your defiant child

your defiant child

8
STEPS TO
BETTER
BEHAVIOR

Russell A. Barkley, PhD
Christine M. Benton

The Guilford Press
New York   London

© 1998 The Guilford Press
A Division of Guilford Publications, Inc.
72 Spring Street, New York, NY 10012
http://www.guilford.com

The information in this volume is not intended as a substitute for consultation with health care professionals. Each individual's health concerns should be evaluated by a qualified professional.

Printed in the United States of America

This book is printed on acid-free paper.

Last digit is print number: 9 8 7 6 5

Library of Congress Cataloging-in-Publication Data

Barkley, Russell A., 1949–
    Your defiant child : eight steps to better behavior / Russell A.
Barkley and Christine M. Benton.
        p.   cm.
    Includes index.
    ISBN 1-57230-405-7 (hc.). — ISBN 1-57230-321-2 (pbk.)
    1. Problem children—Behavior modification.   2. Oppositional
defiant disorder in children.   3. Child rearing.   4. Parenting.
I. Benton, Christine M.   II. Title.
HQ773.B27   1998
649'.64—dc21   98-24231
                                                                          CIP

To Steve Kagen, posthumously, and with deep affection for his courage, strength, kindness, and friendship in the face of one of nature's most cruel, quixotic, and maddening neurological disorders, Tourette syndrome

—R.A.B.

To my parents, Rita and Edward McNesby

—C.M.B.

Preface

This book represents the distillation of more than 20 years of my research on and clinical practice in the nature, causes, and treatment of disruptive behavior problems in children, particularly problems with impulsiveness, hyperactivity, inattention, and defiance. It also draws on thousands of published scientific studies that have focused on these behavior problems and their treatment as reflected in the psychiatric and psychological literature. The child management program contained in this book is one of the most commonly used and effective parent training programs in North America for the management of oppositional and defiant behavior in children. Over the last two decades, I have, through seminars and workshops, introduced more than 10,000 mental health professionals to this program so that they may offer it to families whom they serve in their clinical practices. I also have personally taught more than 2,500 families in this program through my clinical practice.

This research and clinical experience has led me to create a manual for clinical professionals that describes the nature of defiant and oppositional behavior in children, approaches to its assessment, and a highly detailed ten-step program for training parents of these children in more effective ways to reduce conflicts in their relationships with their children. I have also created two professional videotapes on the nature and treatment of defiant children. Although these sources of information appeared to be of great benefit to the professional community that serves clinic-referred children with aggressive, oppositional, and impulsive behavior, they did not give parents direct access to the effective information contained within this program and these resources. I had the growing feeling that only a book written expressly for parents could fill this vastly wider need for direct, useful, no-nonsense information. The eight-step program in this book is an adaptation of the original ten steps, intended to tell parents how they can help their difficult-to-manage children become more agreeable, cooperative, better adjusted, and successful.

My own experience is as an author of scientific research and professional textbooks, so in initial discussions about this book the publisher and I wondered if we could entice Christine Benton to serve as coauthor. Chris had worked with me to make the scientific information I had mastered on attention-deficit/hyperactivity disorder (ADHD) far more interesting, practical, informative, and effective for a general readership in *Taking Charge of ADHD: The Complete, Authoritative Guide for Parents* (New York: Guilford Press, 1995). She agreed, and this book is the result of our mutually satisfying collaboration. If you find this work not only easy to read and digest but also illuminating and even entertaining, all credit goes to Chris. If you find the methods and contents of this program to be at all problematic, then all blame rests with me.

No program of this sort, however, is the work of a single person, or in this case, two people. Several basic pieces of this program were originally developed more than 30 years ago by Constance Hanf, professor emeritas of the Oregon Health Sciences University, who taught them to me during an internship in the care of handicapped children that I had the good fortune to complete at the Child Development and Rehabilitation Center of that fine institution. I am most grateful to her for her sensitive instruction and guidance. The original pieces of her work have since been combined with many other components of effective child management procedures drawn from the works of many other professionals. Several of these people deserve some recognition here for having dedicated their clinical research careers to the study of defiant and aggressive children and their treatment. They are Gerald Patterson, John Reid, Rex Forehand, Robert McMahon, Robert Wahler, Charles Cunningham, Eric Mash, Thomas Dishion, Sheila Eyberg, Carolyn Webster-Stratton, Maureen Forgatch, Mark Roberts, Stephen Hinshaw, William Pelham, James Swanson, Rolf Loeber, and Matthew Sanders. Others whose advice to me over the years has influenced the shape and content of this child management program, thereby improving its effectiveness, are Eric Ward, Mariellen Fischer, Arthur Anastopoulos, George DuPaul, Terri Shelton, Gwen Edwards, Michael Gordon, Maryann Roberts, and Robert Newby, all of whom I have had the honor and pleasure of working with at one time or another. In particular, at times when Chris and I wanted to have recent vignettes of families struggling to cope with and help their defiant children, we turned to Gwen Edwards, chief of the ADHD Clinic at the University of Massachusetts Medical Center, for honest, informative, and engaging anecdotes of real clinical cases. For her assistance in this regard, Chris and I are most grateful.

During the writing of this book, I was partially supported by grants from the National Institute of Mental Health. The contents of this text, however, are solely the responsibility of the authors and do not necessarily represent the official views of nor an implied endorsement by this institute. I am also most grateful to Paul Appelbaum, professor and chairman of the Department of Psychiatry at the University of Massachusetts, for the department's support of me over the last 13 years.

Chris and I both thank Seymour Weingarten and Robert Matloff of The Guilford Press for their encouragement of this project and of our collaboration as its authors, as well as for their continued support of our respective work over many years. We also are grateful for the assistance of the fine production staff at this superlative publishing house. They think of themselves as a family, and we thank them for allowing us to be a small part of it during the course of this project.

Last but never least, Chris and I extend our continuing gratitude to our respective families for their patience with us during this project, for the time it may have stolen from our family lives, and for the education they have given us in the ways of family life with children. We hereby promise to make it up to them. Specifically, thanks are owed to Pat, Steve, and Ken Barkley and to Mike and Liz Benton. Without their support of our efforts and writing, we could never have contemplated, much less undertaken, this work.

Contents

your defiant child

Introduction

When a child acts up all the time, it's easy to believe that he is the only one who behaves that way—or at least that he's the very worst. Naturally, this perception leaves parents berating themselves—"Why can't I control my own child?"—and feeling quite alone.

You are not alone, and quite probably your child's behavior is not worse than that of all the other kids out there. Recent studies show that anywhere from 5 to 8% of American children have a problem with oppositional, noncompliant, and defiant behavior, and those figures include only children whose behavior is bad enough to be diagnosed as a disorder. A great number more could be considered "difficult" (even though their parents might be tempted to call them "impossible").

As you undoubtedly know, these kids drive their parents crazy—and sometimes other adults and even other kids, too—by refusing to do what adults ask or expect of them, by being ornery and temperamental, by breaking or ignoring common rules. As a result, they don't fit in easily or get along with others. The way they act might stand in the way of their succeeding in school and developing a normal social life. Perhaps worst of all, their behavior can seriously harm the parent–child relationship, weakening the bond that all children need to mature into happy and healthy adults.

I know this situation is demoralizing to parents and detrimental to their children because I've counseled thousands of parents who have found themselves trapped in a pattern of power struggles with a son or daughter (most often a son). If you could get together with just a fraction of those parents, you'd realize how many perfectly nice people are facing the same problem you are: loss of control over their children.

This book is my way of offering you the support, experience, and wisdom of other parents. For more than a dozen years, my colleagues and I at the ADHD Clinic, Department of Psychiatry, University of Massachusetts Medical Center in Worcester, Massachusetts, have been training parents, individually and in groups, in methods that help children improve their behavior and get along better in their world. Feedback from parents on what works and what does not has helped us expand and refine our program, so in a very real sense what you will read in this book has been shaped by people like you. Throughout the book, in fact, you will find not only my answers to questions commonly asked by parents over the years but also anecdotes relating how parents—and their kids—have handled difficult situations effectively. I think you'll be as impressed by their creativity as I have been.

Creativity is always an asset in child rearing, but it can't hold a candle to consistency. Consistency in the way you treat your child— the way you set rules, convey expectations, pay attention, encourage good behavior, and impose consequences for bad behavior—is the key to cleaning up your child's act and is therefore the cornerstone of the program in this book. A child with a prickly temperament will always try your patience, and it's only human to get too tired to enforce the rules sometimes, too desperate for control to discipline fairly, too frustrated to keep conflict from escalating. This results in what I call "indiscriminate parenting," and it only makes your child more defiant. Consistency is the way to break that pattern, and it may require a lot of work from you.

Why should the burden of change be on you when it's your child who misbehaves? First of all, your child simply may not be able to change if you don't. Your son or daughter needs help, and you're in a perfect position to give it. Second, a major source of your frustration has been your inability to change your child, try as you might. Most parents actually get relief from taking action in an area where they have ultimate control—their own behavior. Third, you have a lot to gain by making these changes. Up to 80% of the parents who have gone through our program have seen lasting change in their child's behavior. *Children whose defiant behavior is impairing their lives and the lives of their families but is not severe enough to be considered a disorder can achieve normal behavior when their parents make a serious commitment to this program.* Even in more severe cases where a child's defiance persists, the tools learned in this program can greatly reduce the disruptions caused by the child's behavior. When ignored, however, defiant behavior tends to progress into a more debilitating conduct problem in later years.

If your child is over the age of 12 or tends to be very aggressive or violent, please do not undertake this program without the advice of a professional. Defiant behavior is often too deeply entrenched in older children to be resolved solely through self-help; and if your child is violent, a therapist can help you ensure the safety of your whole family. Otherwise, an investment of only a couple of months of concerted effort can help you transform your home from a battleground to a sanctuary by understanding what causes defiant behavior and learning to manage it. As a result, you should be able to improve your child's compliance with your requests and rules and, in turn, restore family harmony.

The book is divided into two parts: "Getting to Know Your Defiant Child" and "Getting Along with Your Defiant Child." Read all about the problem of defiance, what causes it, and the various ways it can be resolved, and by the end of Part One you should have a much firmer idea of what's going on with your child and what you should do about it. Although the book is designed for self-help, some of you may prefer to use it as guided self-help—that is, to find a therapist you feel you can trust and who is familiar with this program and work on it together. Some of you may conclude at the end of Part One that you don't have much of a problem at all. I hope you will read Part Two anyway. It is based on solid, proven child-rearing principles that benefit all children—these principles are enumerated in Chapter 4 at the end of Part One—and I'm sure you'll pick up something useful.

Part Two is the eight-step parent training program. It should take about eight weeks to complete, though you should see significant improvement in your child's behavior and your life in four to six weeks, and you will want to keep using many of the techniques you learn much longer. Each step depends on successful completion of the one before, so please don't skip around or try picking and choosing only the steps that appeal to you. Not everything you'll be asked to do will be fun or easy, but all of it is necessary. *Above all, do not adopt any of the discipline methods that begin in Step 4 (Chapter 8) before completing Steps 1–3.*

The early steps in the program should be a refreshing experience for both you and your child. Because the success of the program depends on reestablishing positive interactions first, you'll start by learning to pay uncritical attention to your child and to praise good behavior—in other words, to catch your child being good. You'll be surprised by how often your child does something that calls for a pat on the back and how much he or she appreciates that you've noticed. Once you have this foundation of cooperation, you can ease your child into the habit of compliance by practicing with little requests that don't tempt the child to balk. Praise is a big but not all-powerful incentive, so your next step is to learn to use rewards as incentives for cooperating more consistently and on tasks your child finds more objectionable.

Only after you've adopted all these positive methods for getting your child to do what he or she needs to do should you move on to the mild, fair disciplinary methods in the program. These include removing rewards for defiance just as you gave them for compliance, as well as using time-out effectively. By this point in the program (following Step 5), you should have made significant strides, but if you need help controlling your child's behavior away from home, Steps 6 and 7 offer techniques for extending these methods to public places and to school. Part Two ends with a look ahead—how to sustain the progress you've made and how to anticipate and handle future behavior problems.

At the end of the book are some resources for additional information and support. Remember, though, that there are many caring, competent professionals available to help you if this book is not enough. Please contact one—starting with your pediatrician—if you need further assistance.

PART ONE

Getting to Know
Your Defiant Child

CHAPTER 1

Is Something Wrong with My Child?

It's frightening and painful to suspect that something is wrong with your child. When the cause of your worry is your child's misbehavior, especially toward you, it's confusing and exhausting, too. On the one hand, you believe that *no one* else your child's age acts like that . . . but on the other, don't all kids disobey and challenge parental authority? Don't they all go through phases? Do you really have anything to be concerned about at all? You're probably losing sleep agonizing over questions like these. And that's the last thing you need if you usually spend your days battling with your child.

In this chapter, I hope to help you start rebuilding the strength you need to address the problems you're experiencing with your son or daughter, with the ultimate goal of restoring the precious relationship we all want and deserve to have with our children. Let's begin answering the question that's probably keeping you awake at night— "Is something wrong with my child?"—through a simple test. Answer "never or rarely," "sometimes," "often," "or very often" (and save your answers for later comparison).

My child . . .

1. Loses his/her temper

Never or rarely   Sometimes   Often   Very often

2. Argues with adults

Never or rarely   Sometimes   Often   Very often

3. *Actively defies or refuses to comply with adults' requests or rules*

Never or rarely   Sometimes   Often   Very often

4. *Deliberately annoys people*

Never or rarely   Sometimes   Often   Very often

5. *Blames others for his or her mistakes or misbehavior*

Never or rarely   Sometimes   Often   Very often

6. *Is touchy or easily annoyed by others*

Never or rarely   Sometimes   Often   Very often

7. *Is angry and resentful*

Never or rarely   Sometimes   Often   Very often

8. *Is spiteful or vindictive*

Never or rarely   Sometimes   Often   Very often

If you answered "often" or "very often" to at least four of these questions, your concerns are probably well founded. Your child's behavior may be a sign of a legitimate problem, and you're doing the right thing by reading this book. Generalizing may not, however, give you a completely satisfactory answer. To know where your child stands, you probably need to take a closer look at the pattern of his or her behavior. Where and when does your child act out? How severe is the misbehavior you see? How does it compare to what other kids do and say?

If the quiz was too broad to describe your child accurately, maybe the following scenarios will strike a familiar chord:

• "Jenny's a loving, affectionate girl, and her teachers say she's very bright, but ask her to do something she doesn't want to do and watch out. It's like she becomes a different child—loud, hostile, and downright nasty. The more I try to explain that whether she goes to bed on time, puts away her toys, or brushes her teeth is not up to her, the louder she shouts 'No!' at us. She just doesn't seem to get it."

• "Ben just can't behave anywhere. I've had to drag him out of toy stores and ended up in shouting matches over the candy he insists on having at the grocery store. I've gotten to the point where I do everything I can to stay home. I just don't have the energy to deal with crisis after crisis, day in and day out."

- "I can see that Josh is getting depressed and withdrawn, but I just don't know what to do. I've tried to explain to him that of course no one wants to play with him when he's so bossy. He just can't have his own way all the time. When he was the only one on the block who wasn't invited to Billy's birthday party, it broke my heart."

- "I feel like I'm on one of those wheels they put in hamsters' cages, and I don't know how to get off. Annie talks back, and I yell. She yells back, and I yell louder. I threaten punishment, and she still doesn't obey. I get madder and madder until I either scare myself or get exhausted. That's when I start to back down, and before I know it I've wasted 20 minutes arguing with a 5-year-old without getting her to do what I've asked. "

- "I was so thrown by Susie's calm refusal to do what she was told that I actually took her to the ear doctor for special tests. That she couldn't hear me was the only logical reason I could come up with for her ignoring me so often."

- "Frankie's always had a temper, always had a real mind of his own. We didn't worry too much about it when he was two—just shook our heads and told ourselves he'd outgrow it. But now we've watched all the other kids leave the 'terrible twos' and move on, and at age six Frankie still throws tantrums every day, still grabs the other kids' toys, pushes and shoves to be first in line, and has to be literally wrestled into bed every night. How much longer is this going to last?"

The common thread running through these parental laments is *defiance*. Call it resistance, opposition, contrariness, disobedience, willfulness, sass, freshness, or any of a dozen other terms, it's the repeated failure of a child to follow rules, obey commands or comply with requests, and generally do what parents, teachers, peers, and society at large expect children to do. Recognizing your child in one or more of the preceding descriptions may give you a little more to go on, but it still may not be enough to tell you whether something is wrong. Oppositional, defiant behavior can take a perplexing variety of forms, and parents define "misbehavior" in many different ways, depending on how they expect children to behave and how well they tolerate any behavior that falls outside those limits. Therefore, to answer the question, "Is there really anything *wrong*, or is it just me?" you need some reliable objective measures. My colleagues and I consider a child oppositional and defiant when the child demonstrates a pattern of these three types of behavior:

1. The child fails to start doing what you ask within one minute after you make the request (or one minute following the point at which you say the child has to do what you ask, such as after the cartoon he is watching is over).

2. The child fails to finish what you've asked her to do. Some children may get up and start making their beds as requested right away, but then they run off to do something more appealing in the middle of the chore.

3. The child violates rules of conduct already taught. Does your son know that swearing is unacceptable in your house, but he does it anyway? Does your daughter understand the rule "no snacks without permission" but constantly take food from the refrigerator without asking? Noncompliant and defiant behavior is most likely to appear at home or in public, but your child may also be acting out at school, leaving his desk in class without permission or talking throughout a teacher's lecture.

One of the most problematic aspects of identifying defiant behavior in children, both for their parents and for psychologists, is that these three types of behavior *can* take so many forms and that they appear with widely varying degrees of aggression. Some kids, like Susie above, are pretty passive in their avoidance of requests and rules. Others, perhaps Jenny and Frankie, might express their defiance very vocally, even physically. Many parents report that their children shout and swear at them or even hit or push them when asked to do something they don't want to do. Oppositional, defiant behavior can run the gamut from whining, complaining, and crying to arguing, yelling, screaming, and swearing. It may range from simply drifting away from chores to destroying property and getting into fights. Maybe you've seen some of these tendencies in your child:

Oppositional, defiant children . . .
- Change from content to angry in a second.
- Fight the inevitable, such as going to bed, going to school, or

coming to the table at mealtimes, even when they know that eventually they'll be forced to comply.
- Insist on having their own way when playing with friends.
- Argue as vociferously about performing the little tasks as the big ones, as long as it's something they don't want to do.
- May lie or cheat to escape responsibility for their actions.
- Like to "get back at" people instead of forgetting about minor slights.
- Are easily irritated.
- May seem hostile toward particular people for no obvious reason.
- Ignore commands.
- Deliberately disobey their parents and sometimes other adults.
- Break rules indiscriminately.
- Badger or taunt people, apparently for fun.
- Resist interrupting play.
- Seem to have a chip on their shoulder.
- Can't control their temper as well as other children of their age.
- Often break or destroy things out of anger.
- May indulge in self-destructive behavior such as holding their breath or banging their head.
- Show little respect or regard for their parents, especially Mom.

If all of this is beginning to paint a pretty accurate picture of your child, read on. This chapter tells you what else you need to know about your child's behavior to determine whether you have a bona fide problem to be solved or just a phase to be endured. It explains how and when defiance is diagnosed as a disorder and what other problems may accompany it. In the following pages, you'll gain an understanding of how severe your child's problem might be and whether you need help beyond this book. Most of you, however, will be reassured to discover that you don't need professional help to manage this problem. In fact, the more you learn about the nature of defiance in children, the less you'll view it as "something wrong with your child" and the more you'll see it as a difficult situation with highly workable solutions. I trust you'll finish this chapter with new hope that you can meet this challenge, that you can restore the loving relationship with your child that you both deserve, and that this problem does not have to stand in the way of your child's achieving a happy, healthy adulthood.

When Does a Phase Become a Problem?

No matter how many times you answered "often" in the test at the beginning of this chapter, if these behaviors are a relatively recent development, you might not have any reason to be concerned. Even a week of "No, I won't!" can seem like eternity, but the fact is that unless this behavior has been going on for at least six months, it may prove temporary. How do you know, and what might be going on in that case?

As horrifying as it may seem, what your child is doing may be completely normal—for his or her age. You shouldn't consider an 18- or 24-month-old abnormally defiant just because she says "no" to everything. Nor would I say that nine-year-old Harry had a disorder just because the nice third-grader has turned into a belligerent, rule-breaking fourth-grader—so have all his classmates. Perhaps you need only hang in there, as parents do during other trying phases, such as the "terrible twos" and the "torturous teens."

A 5-year-old who says "no" to everything like someone half his age, however, is another story, and so is the 12-year-old who continues her immature practice of throwing tantrums when asked to do something that doesn't appeal to her. In these cases, you have to look at the child's pattern of behavior throughout childhood. Some children show signs of difficult temperament from a very early age, so their parents aren't so much surprised as dismayed when difficult turns into defiant.

When the behavior is brand-new, though, you have to consider the possibility that some other factor is causing the child's defiance. Children may "act out" in response to everything from puberty to moving to their parents' divorce. Defiant behavior may be their expression of stress caused by a parent or sibling's illness, a parent's extended business trip, or a new baby in the family. A prolonged illness of his own could throw the behavior of your normally even-tempered son out of kilter, just as passing a developmental milestone can wreak havoc with the "attitude" of your formerly cooperative daughter. The key is the duration of the behavior. We have found that the stress of a single event usually resolves itself within six months, so new defiant behavior generally should not be cause for alarm unless it lasts longer than that. When it does, you need to determine whether an ongoing stressor is at work. If you know that something in your child's environment continues to weigh on the child emotionally—strife between parents, a major change in family lifestyle, and so forth—you may want to seek counseling. Anytime your child demonstrates an abrupt, radical change in personality, you should get a medical opinion. See Chapter 3 for advice on obtaining professional help.

You also may want to seek help if you notice other symptoms along with your child's defiance. Some defiant children also have attention-deficit/hyperactivity disorder (ADHD). Although you may be able to manage the child's defiance with the help of this book, you'll want the advice of a professional on ADHD; again, see Chapter 3. As you'll learn in Chapter 2, other problems also can accompany defiance, including depression—here, too, you'll want a professional evaluation.

Even if you've determined that your child's defiant behavior may very well be a passing phase, an evil necessity of development, or a temporary condition, do read through the principles and techniques in Chapters 4–12, paying particular attention to accentuating the positive in your child. There's no point in letting temporary conflict create a permanent rift between you and your child, so remember to emphasize incentives over punishment, to pay attention to the acceptable behavior your child displays, and to build some form of pleasant time together into every day. And always do something about it if you find your child's behavior is wreaking havoc in your family. I've found that the program laid out in Part Two can make any defiant phase pass much more smoothly. Try it if you think taking action will give you peace of mind and restore a modicum of tranquillity to your home.

When Does "Difficult" Become "Disorder"?

Let's assume your child's behavior fits the profile for defiance that we've drawn so far, it has continued unabated, and you know of no external stressor in your child's life. Does this mean something is seriously wrong with your son or daughter? Do you need to rush your child off to a psychologist, psychiatrist, or pediatrician for diagnosis and treatment? Not necessarily.

Unless you answered "often" or "very often" to six or more of the questions in the preceding test or your child is prone to violence, you probably don't need a professional diagnosis or professional help. Except in severe cases, where the child is greatly impaired by the defiant behavior, affixing a clinical label to your child's problem may not have any practical purpose. We all know adults who are called "high-strung" or "demanding" or "rigid." We may not find them easy to deal with, but we chalk that up to temperament. It may be perfectly feasible for you to view your child this way.

If you're not comfortable leaving it at that, the only reliable way to know the difference between a child with a difficult temperament and one with a psychological disorder is to have the child undergo a professional evaluation by a qualified psychologist or psychiatrist. If your child's problem *is* severe, this evaluation can identify any intertwined disorders—such as ADHD—and ensure that your child gets the necessary treatment for other problems that often accompany a behavioral disorder. Otherwise, you can go a long way toward improving your child's life and yours with self-help such as the program in this book. In fact, even in severe cases this self-help program can be of great use, perhaps in conjunction with professional therapy.

In Chapter 2, I explain why the causes of defiance often make it receptive to pretty simple treatment without drugs or psychotherapy. The main thing the program in this book requires is your diligence, your parental commitment to applying the recommended principles and techniques consistently.

Some parents, of course, simply rest more easily after they have gotten the advice of an expert. If you choose that route, be aware that you won't find consensus within the professional community on how and when to diagnose noncompliance/defiance as a true disorder. What mental health professionals call *oppositional defiant disorder* (ODD) is really a set of behaviors, and behaviors are difficult to measure. That may be why some scientists believe that in order to diagnose and treat a behavioral problem as a disorder, a "harmful dysfunction" must be identified, and a harmful dysfunction should be defined in part by the presence of an "aberration in an internal, normal mental or cognitive mechanism." In other words, a troublesome behavior pattern, some believe, is not enough; there must be something organically "wrong" with the child to justify diagnosing and treating the behavior as a disorder.

No one has identified a specific physical dysfunction that causes defiant behavior, but that does not mean that many psychologists, including my colleagues and me, will not treat the problem. We believe it simply causes too much distress to ignore. It does mean, however, that we must rely on how the child acts in determining whether a disorder exists.

As already mentioned, the problem with measuring behavior is that so many factors are involved. A child's behavior at any given moment will be determined not only by internal factors—temperament, health, memory, and others—but also by an almost infinite number of factors in the environment. Another complication is, as behavioral psychologists will explain, that virtually all behavior can be considered normal. Because behavior is almost always relative, it's degree that matters—how frequent, how constant, and how severe the child's defiance is.

One way to evaluate any aspect of any child's behavior is to picture it as falling somewhere on a continuum. With one end of the line representing the least possible amount of a behavior and the other the greatest possible amount, you could plot how talkative your child is, how quick-tempered, shy, active, or impulsive. Where your child's behavior falls on that line gives you an idea of how close to "average" or "normal" the child's behavior is based on the range of behavior for all children. If you picture such a continuum for defiance, a psychologist's evaluation will essentially be an attempt to see where your child's behavior falls on that line. Chances are, if you believe your child's behavior is problematic enough to warrant a professional opinion, the evaluation will determine that your child's defiance falls pretty far to the extreme end for that behavior (although it may not, for reasons discussed on page 17).

To determine where a child falls on the continuum, scientists have come up with various rating scales, such as the simple one at the beginning of this chapter. To receive a diagnosis of oppositional defiant disorder, a child must fall above the 93rd percentile for a standardized behavior rating scale designed for this purpose. Children who fall between the 84th and 93rd percentiles are often said to have "borderline" cases of the disorder.

Three criteria that help clinicians place children on the defiant-behavior continuum—that tell them something about the degree of the child's defiance—are the *constancy, frequency,* and *severity* of the behavior. You've probably already established the criterion of *constancy*—your child has been acting like this for at least six months. To measure *frequency* and *severity,* complete the following questionnaire.

DEFIANCE IN VARIOUS HOME SITUATIONS

If your child disobeys or defies your instructions, commands, or rules in any of the following situations, circle *Yes,* then circle the number that reflects how severe the problem is for you. If not, circle *No.* Then add up the *Yes* answers you circled and calculate the average severity rating. Save your answers for later comparison.

Situations	*Yes/No*		*Mild*								*Severe*
While playing alone	Yes	No	1	2	3	4	5	6	7	8	9
While playing with other children	Yes	No	1	2	3	4	5	6	7	8	9
At mealtimes	Yes	No	1	2	3	4	5	6	7	8	9
Getting dressed	Yes	No	1	2	3	4	5	6	7	8	9
Washing and bathing	Yes	No	1	2	3	4	5	6	7	8	9
While you are on the phone	Yes	No	1	2	3	4	5	6	7	8	9
While watching TV	Yes	No	1	2	3	4	5	6	7	8	9
When visitors are in your home	Yes	No	1	2	3	4	5	6	7	8	9
While visiting someone else	Yes	No	1	2	3	4	5	6	7	8	9
In public (restaurants, stores, church, etc.)	Yes	No	1	2	3	4	5	6	7	8	9
When father is home	Yes	No	1	2	3	4	5	6	7	8	9
When asked to do chores	Yes	No	1	2	3	4	5	6	7	8	9

When asked to do homework	Yes	No		1	2	3	4	5	6	7	8	9
At bedtime	Yes	No		1	2	3	4	5	6	7	8	9
While in the car	Yes	No		1	2	3	4	5	6	7	8	9
When with a babysitter	Yes	No		1	2	3	4	5	6	7	8	9

Total number of problem situations _____   Mean severity score _____

If your frustration with your child sometimes pushes you to exaggeration ("How often does Jenny argue with adults? Try *constantly*"), this form may give you a slightly more accurate view of your child's defiance. Perhaps out of the 16 situations listed, your child really has a problem with noncompliance in only 5. Maybe your child causes a problem in most of the settings, but it's a mild problem. Whatever you learn through this process, it probably will become clear that you're facing a problem that can be broken down into manageable segments rather than the relentless harassment that living with a defiant child can feel like. One handicap that all such scales have is that they are based on the perceptions of observers, which are not always unfailingly objective. As already stated, your perception of your child's misbehavior is colored by your expectations and your own temperament. Every week my colleagues and I see at least a few parents whose children fall pretty squarely in the middle of the continuum for defiant behavior. The only problem turns out to be the parents' exaggerated concern about their children's adjustment and their own parental competence, distortions that feel quite accurate but are based on unrealistic expectations of both the children and themselves. I determine this just as often through personal interviews as through questionnaires and rating scales. You, too, can check your perceptions by seeing whether they jibe with those of others who spend time around your child. Are neighbors, relatives, and friends giving you feedback that your child's behavior is more inappropriate or unacceptable than normal for the child's age and gender? Has a preschool teacher, babysitter, or other child-care worker commented to you that your child is considerably more difficult to manage than other children? If so, you know you're not totally off the mark. If it turns out you're the only one who sees your child as abnormally defiant, you have a couple of options: (1) seek help for yourself—or the simple reassurance that I usually provide that everything is fine—from a professional, and/or (2) go ahead and adopt some of the program from Part Two of this book. It's based on solid child-rearing principles that can help all families, and you may find that the simple act of having a plan to fall back on is enough to calm you down.

All of the tools I've provided—the short questionnaires and interview-type questions, the profiles, and the other resources to consult—are intended to help you organize your thoughts at a time when emotion and stress may be tossing logic to the wind. Hopefully, you've gained a little confidence by injecting a measure of science into your evaluation of your child. I firmly believe that no one knows children like their own parents, so you're probably right to trust your own preliminary conclusions about whether something is wrong. If you still have doubts, take a close look at what type of damage is being done by your child's behavior.

When Do You Need to Take Action?

Now that you have a lot of indicators to tell you whether your child is likely abnormally defiant or noncompliant, I can state unequivocally that the most important indicator of all is how the behavior is affecting your child and others. If you answer "yes" to the following two sets of questions, you'll gain much from following the program in this book, even if you answered "often" to fewer than four of the questions in the test at the beginning of this chapter.

1. Is your child significantly impaired by the defiant/noncompliant behavior? Is your son unable to take care of himself as he should for his age (hygiene, dressing, and the like)? Does your daughter fail to do chores and homework considered reasonable for her age? Does your child have trouble getting along with other kids and following rules in your absence compared with other kids of that age? If your child can't function in these ways as would be expected for his or her intelligence level, impairment certainly exists.

2. Is your child's defiant behavior causing emotional distress to the child and—even more likely—to you, as well as to siblings and peers? If your child has experienced significant anger, unhappiness, or distress much of the day for at least two weeks, you should be alerted to a problem. Does your son or daughter seem anxious, depressed, or withdrawn? What about you? If you're losing your days in a blur of daily battles, losing your sanity in an increasingly futile effort to bend your child's will to your own, something is obviously wrong. Do you feel demoralized, as if you never do anything right anymore? Are you starting to avoid interactions with your child altogether, abdicating parenthood at some level? Are you losing sleep, feeling depressed, angry, or resentful? It's time to do something about the problem.

There are other compelling reasons as well for taking action now.

1. Defiance seems to be on the rise among children today. That is the impression among my colleagues, and it is supported by a recent study conducted at the University of Vermont in which two generations of children from around the state were surveyed.

HOW COMMON IS DEFIANCE IN CHILDREN?

The information available on the prevalence of defiance among children is limited to those with ODD and CD, as defined by the American Psychiatric Association's *Diagnostic and Statistical Manual of Mental Disorders* (DSM). This book lists diagnostic criteria for diagnosing various psychiatric disorders in an attempt to standardize the clinical process of diagnosing mental, emotional, and behavioral problems that affect adults and children. Unfortunately, because the studies conducted have been based on different editions of the DSM, they do not all define ODD and CD in the same way. Nor have they all studied children of the same ages. Therefore, the figures vary pretty widely. Clearly, too, there are even more children than the following rates suggest who have defiance that is not severe enough to be diagnosed as ODD or CD.

• ***How many children have ODD?*** The fourth edition of the DSM, DSM-IV (Washington, DC: American Psychiatric Association, 1994), re-

(cont.)

ports that anywhere from 2 to 16% of American children have ODD and that CD affects the same percentages. One study of 1,096 6- to 17-year-olds found 4.9% with ODD. Another study, on 931 5- to 14-year-old boys, showed 3.2% with ODD, but because the study was based solely on teacher ratings and because most defiance appears at home and in public rather than at school, those findings may be deceptively low. A large study of 11-year-olds found 5.7% with ODD. Among adolescents, studies have reported 1.7 to 2.5% with ODD.

• **How many children have CD?** Although DSM-IV reported that the same percentage of children (2 to 16%) have CD as have ODD, most studies show that a significantly lower percentage have CD than ODD: 1.9% of 6- to 17-year-olds with CD compared to 4.9 percent with ODD; 1.3 percent of 5- to 14-year-olds with CD compared to 3.2% with ODD; 3.4% of 11-year-olds with CD compared to 5.7% with ODD. However, the study of teenagers found 3.2 to 7.3% with CD compared to 1.7 to 2.5% with ODD. Why does the rate of ODD go down and the rate of CD go up in adolescence? Probably because some children grow out of their defiance by that time, *whereas others progress into CD.*

• **Are boys more likely to be defiant than girls?** Yes, according to a great majority of studies. DSM-IV reported that 6 to 16% of boys had CD compared to only 2 to 9% of girls. Among the 11-year-olds studied (see the preceding paragraph), the male-to-female ratio for ODD was 2.2 to 1; for CD, it was 3.2 to 1. Among teenagers, the male-to-female ratio fell between two to one and three to one for both ODD and CD, though one review has suggested that girls may catch up to boys in the rate of CD by adolescence.

2. ODD is the most common early developmental stage for later progression into conduct disorder (CD), which is a more severe form of oppositional behavior that often appears during adolescence. (The criteria for CD are listed in the Appendix.)

3. Over time ODD causes increasing conflict within the family and elsewhere. Defiance that is allowed to continue almost always gets worse. Like a glacier, it rolls relentlessly over the landscape of a family's life, damaging family and social relationships, gouging chunks out of the self-esteem of parents and child, destroying peace and tranquillity at home. As defiance continues, so does family conflict and the antisocial attitude of the child. In turn, these lead to a downward spiral by which the parents feel powerless, the whole family loses its affection for each other and starts to avoid shared activities, and the family becomes isolated from the larger social world as well. When defiance continues unabated, you can end up depressed, stressed out, and demoralized; problems often arise between the parents, because defiance typically appears more often between the child and one parent than between the child and the other. Finally, siblings, who often get short shrift from their parents when a defiant child is preoccupying Mom and Dad, can end up hostile and resentful toward the defiant child and the parents.

4. Conflicts between parent and child become an entrenched form of interaction that worsens with time. In any given interaction, the parent issues a command or request. When the child doesn't comply, the parent repeats the command several more times, to no avail. The parent then threatens the child, often a few times. When that doesn't work either, the parent either acquiesces or exacts some punishment—in extreme cases becoming physically aggressive. Acquiescence, of course, only reinforces the child's behavior, teaching the child that he or she can get out of anything as long as the child persists in refusing to comply. The parents, too, become so accustomed to this pattern that they often fail to provide positive reinforcement for the times when the child does cooperate, inadvertently teaching the child further that compliance is undesirable.

5. Many children simply don't outgrow this problem. Evidence shows that childhood defiance or aggressiveness may, in fact, be one of the most stable of childhood behavioral disorders across development. This means intervention is necessary.

6. Defiant behavior very often leads to later adjustment problems. The stubbornness, temper outbursts, defiance, arguing, irritability, and blaming that begin at ages 4 through 6 eventually give way to disruptive acts like bullying, vandalism, truancy, and running away by age 9 or 10. Untreated children may, as teens, turn to criminal activity and substance abuse. They perform poorly academically and are not well accepted by their peers. They are at higher risk than others for depression and suicide attempts.

If you think about it, you have to admit that much of what your child faces in the future will require some form of compliance. Imagine the disabilities of a child who isn't toilet-trained because he can't heed his parents' requests; the disadvantage of a child who is struggling academically but can't sit down with his parents to get help with homework and studying. How will your child fit into the world if she alienates everyone she encounters? Picture the limited world of a child who is barred from participation in Scouts, banned from museums, and thrown out of Little League.

Now picture the prickly son or daughter you see before you transforming with maturation into a well-adjusted, well-liked, confident young adult. It's not too late, but much depends on you. I'll explain why in the next chapter.

RECAP: THE PROBLEM

Defiance is a distressing behavior problem that takes many forms but is defined in general by a child's failure to comply with commands and requests, to follow through on assigned tasks, and to follow rules clearly learned and understood. It can make your life difficult, and therefore it warrants some kind of corrective action when it lasts longer than six months, is not related to a developmental phase or temporary stressor, is relatively severe, and has a strong negative effect on your child and your family.

You can get a good idea of how severe your child's problem is and what type of action it demands from you by using the forms and questionnaires in this chapter. Noncompliant, defiant behavior that falls toward the extreme end of the continuum may be diagnosable as oppositional defiant disorder (ODD) or conduct disorder (CD), but your child's life and yours may benefit from the child management/parent training program in Part Two of this book even if your child's problem is less severe. Though some kids do outgrow defiance, the sizable number that do not often progress to the more serious conduct disorder, and family conflict definitely increases when a child's defiance persists. If this chapter has helped you identify a significant behavior problem in your child, you will want to act now to protect your child's future and the health and happiness of your home and family.

CHAPTER 2

Why Is This Happening to My Family?

When a child's defiance begins to terrorize your household, it's very tempting to look for someone to blame. Throwing up your hands and proclaiming, "Jimmy is just a monster," or "I guess I'm just a terrible parent," may even offer a little relief from the anxiety of asking yourself, "*Why?*" But as you probably know, it's a fleeting comfort, because what you really need is answers that you can use to make things better. What you really want is some assurance that your child isn't a hopeless case and you're not a total failure.

You'll find both well-researched answers and plenty of reassurance in this chapter. The most important fundamental facts that we have about defiant behavior are that (1) it takes time to develop and (2) it arises from a complicated set of causes. So don't be too hard on yourself if you haven't been able to figure out how you and your child got where you are today. In the following pages, I break down what we know into manageable segments that will help you take a clearer look at what's been happening at home. As you read, please remember that there's only one purpose for the clarity of hindsight I hope you'll gain in this chapter: to illuminate the future.

Behavior Never Occurs in a Vacuum

Ten-year-old Cindy and her mother had spent the last hour happily working together on a trail map they were supposed to take to Cindy's Girl Scout meeting that evening. When Mom handed Cindy a marker to use for the lake-side trail, just as she had been doing for the other trails drawn, Cindy sudden-ly pushed the pen back at her mother and shouted, "No! You do it!" Mom looked up at Cindy in surprise and said, "Why? We agreed you would do all the drawing." Cindy's voice got even louder: "I said no!" She then stood up, glared at her mother, slapped her hard on the arm, and stomped out of the room.

The Simmons family was in the middle of a typical dinner. Eight-year-old Sam, famished after an afternoon of soccer practice, was happily wolfing down his chicken, slowing down only when his mother quietly reminded him that the food wasn't going anywhere. Twelve-year-old Tina was telling her parents about that day's science test in between bites. Ten-year-old Brian, noisily rocking back and forth in his chair, roughly pushed his food around on his plate until most of it ended up on his lap or the floor. Each time he bent to retrieve it, he took the opportunity to jab his brother in the side with his elbow. Despite Sam's increasingly annoyed protests, Mom and Dad studiously ig-nored Brian's antics.

It was 8:30, nine-year-old Tim's weeknight bedtime, and the battle had begun. As usual, Tim's mother firmly told him to turn off the TV and brush his teeth. Also as usual, Tim ignored her. She raised her voice; he didn't budge. She marched over to the TV and turned it off; he turned it back on. And so it went, Tim's mother planting herself between her son and the TV, bodily lift-ing him to his feet and pointing him toward the bathroom, the verbal battle es-calating with each passing minute until finally, at 9:30, Tim fell tearfully into bed and his mother fell dejectedly into an armchair.

No wonder you're ready to throw up your hands. When children behave this way, it's hard to see any rhyme or reason in their actions. Why would Cindy suddenly refuse to cooperate with her mother, de-spite apparently having enjoyed the project to that point? Why does Brian behave so differently from his siblings, despite all three having apparently reasonable parents? Why does Tim pull the same antibed-time tricks every night when he has plenty of proof that bedtime is in-evitable?

When children behave in ways that run counter to our expecta-tions, we are baffled. But the fact that any individual incident is beyond our immediate understanding doesn't mean that the child is be-having at random. In any given situation, how your child behaves (how *any* child behaves) is a function of many factors, among them the child's innate personality and temperament, the child's learning histo-ry within the family, and the immediate consequences at hand. How these factors shake out in a particular situation may never be entirely predictable, but having some idea of what is involved in your child's behavior will at least release you from the paralysis of total confusion.

As her mother will tell you, Cindy has always had a hard time controlling her impulses. When she starts to get bored with a project, she wants it to end . . . *now.* Where other kids might stick it out, Cindy strikes out. She's learned over the years that pleading and arguing don't always get her what she wants but hitting nearly always makes people back down.

Brian acts differently from his siblings because he *is* different. He can't sit still long enough to listen to the soft voice of reason that works with Sam and Tina, and ignoring him doesn't discourage his misbehavior because he's not doing it for attention—he's doing it be-cause he has no strong incentive to stop. Even more motivating, how-ever, is that he gets out of a meal he doesn't like and a chance to return to his beloved Sega games.

As for Tim, sure he knows that bedtime is inevitable. He just doesn't care. Because he has a hard time looking ahead, his only goal is to put off what he finds unappealing right now. Any postponement of the inevitable is a victory to him.

All of this is easy for me to say—I've been observing these chil-dren for quite some time from the safe emotional distance that a par-ent rarely has. If you could see your child the way I've been able to see Cindy, Brian, and Tim, you too would recognize various forces at work in the child's behavior:

1. There's the child's temperament and other characteristics. Cindy is extremely bright but also irritable and hot-tempered. Brian is highly active and tends to hold grudges against those who annoy him (especially his little brother, who earlier that day had broken Brian's favorite car). Tim is generally cheerful but resists any change that isn't his own idea and doesn't seem to be able to look beyond this moment in time.

2. Then there's the history of your interactions with your child.
Over time children gather a wealth of information in their mental
archives: how far they can push you, what gets a reaction and what
does not, what they get for being "good" as well as what they get for
being "bad," and much, much more. And it is especially what they get
out of, escape from, or avoid doing when they act this way that is so
critical to understanding their behavior. A major goal of growing children is to make their world sensible and predictable. You, as a parent,
are a huge part of that world, and how you talk to and treat your child
teaches him how to behave with you as surely as Pavlov taught his
dog. A couple of times Cindy's mother was so distressed by her
daughter's physical aggression that she gave her what she wanted,
and that was enough to convince Cindy that hitting was the way to go.
Brian has learned that he can torture his brother relentlessly because
his parents believe that if they keep ignoring it, he'll outgrow it. Tim
knows that if he keeps fighting her, he'll be able to avoid whatever his
mother wants him to do for quite a while.

3. Then there's your personality. Cindy's mother is very reasonable and logical; she's totally thrown by Cindy's outbursts of temper.
Brian's parents both have a low threshold for excitement; their middle
child's "personality" distresses them so severely that they've begun to
retreat from him altogether. Tim and his mother are like two peas in a
pod—both prickly and demanding, both rigid and immature for their
age.

4. Finally, there are all the other bits of your family's environment.
Events, relationships, and situations inside and outside the home can
affect a child's behavior. Both Cindy and her mother are hurting over a
bitter divorce and custody battle. Brian's father has severe asthma,
which makes both parents very anxious. Tim's mother is struggling to
make ends meet, exhausted by the demands of working during the
day and going to school in the evening.

Take another look at your situation: How would you describe
your child's temperament? Can you step back and see what motivates
her in various circumstances? Can you identify a pattern in the way
the two of you act when you ask your child to do something or stop
doing something—or when your child asks you for something? How
would you describe yourself? Are you generally as cool as a cucumber

or as hot as a chili pepper? Do you have the patience of a saint or the world's shortest fuse? Are you and your child very different or very similar? What about the rest of your life—tranquil or crazed, manageable or loaded with stress? It's difficult to see ourselves and our loved ones with crystal clarity, so a little farther on I provide some tools to help you explore these factors one at a time. One of the reasons we all have trouble sorting out the many factors involved in behavior is that they're intertwined in complex ways.

Every Action Has an Equal— and Opposite!—Reaction

Not only does each of these factors shape your child's behavior, but each affects all the others—and back again. Your child's irritability affects your mood, and your bad mood makes the child more defensive and defiant. Your poor health makes you testy, which encourages your child to oppose you, which puts more stress on you and worsens your health. You can watch this merry-go-round spinning within individual confrontations and also over long stretches of time. Let's say Tim's mother, exhausted by the stress of being her family's sole support, has no energy to control her angry responses to her ever-demanding child. Tim's "difficult personality" eventually becomes diagnosable ODD. With additional stress and less rest, Tim's mother ends up suffering from chronic headaches. After missing too many days of work due to pain, she loses her job and is now in dire financial straits. This stress worsens the interactions between Mom and Tim, and Tim begins to have run-ins with the law. Now that Mom has to add lawyers' bills to an ever-growing pile of commitments she can't meet, you can imagine where the mother–son relationship is headed.

What Do You Think Causes Your Child's Defiance?

Many of the families I counsel have the deck stacked against them: A child who is temperamental and impulsive, with a high activity level and a short attention span, is being reared by parents who have a lot of the same characteristics, as well as marital, financial, and other forms of stress, and who are unsure of how to act in encounters with their defiant child. Once they realize how complex the causes of defiance can be, they're a lot less quick to look for a convenient scapegoat to explain the problem. With temperament a fixed element and many life stresses out of one's control as well, defiance can't really be called anyone's fault, can it?

What about you? What do *you* think causes your child to be defiant? Answer the following questions. If you live together, have the child's other parent answer them separately.

1. Imagine a typical confrontation with your child. What makes the child refuse to comply with your wishes in individual cases like those? What seems to motivate the child? What does the child expect to get out of acting this way?

2. Now list the influences you believe might be at work—the child's makeup, your (and your spouse's) temperament, your (and your spouse's) approach to dealing with the child, and events and circumstances affecting the family.

3. How long has the child's behavior toward you (and possibly others) been defiant, noncompliant, or oppositional? When did it first become a problem?

Between you and your child's other parent, you may very well see a glimmering of a problem in each of the four factors that contribute to defiance. Even if you're luckier in life than most of my patients, you'll want to explore the causes further. Remember that over time, little problems can add up to a pretty sizable problem of defiant behavior. But once you know what is at work, you can try to change the factors you have power over and try to work around those you don't.

The Child: Biology, Environment, or a Little of Each?

When I ask parents what they think causes their child's defiance, I get a pretty broad range of answers. Generally, though, the answers break down into "nature versus nurture" explanations: Either the child was destined to be this way by biology or something in the child's environment is to blame. In 40 to 60% or more of all cases, defiant children have some inborn characteristic that makes them prone to oppositional behavior. But as you'll see, trying to isolate biology from environment is a lot like trying to get a better look at the design in a rich tapestry by pulling the threads apart. You want to understand which of your child's characteristics might contribute to defiance—not to attach some label to the child but to understand better what makes the child tick: What motivates her? How does he think? What will he feel like in different situations? What bothers her most? What are her strengths?

Temperament or "Personality"

Some children simply seem to be troubled and troublesome from birth, starting life with poor eating and sleeping habits, a tendency to be overactive and oversensitive, and a leaning toward irritability, moodiness, and fussiness. As many parents attest, these signs of "difficult" temperament are easily recognizable as early as a baby's first six months. Did your child cry when overstimulated as an infant? Did a slight change in routine throw her off and make her moody for days, even weeks? Was he "colicky"? What about now? Is the child overly fastidious, rigid, moody, easily angered, or flighty?

Like behavior, your child's temperament can be seen as falling somewhere along a continuum. To find your child's niche on that line, rate the different problem traits you see in your child on a severity scale of 1 to 10 (1 = no problem or a very rare problem, 5 = a moderate problem or one that occurs often, 10 = a serious problem or one that almost always occurs).

PROFILE OF YOUR CHILD'S TEMPERAMENT

Problems with impulse control:

1   2   3   4   5   6   7   8   9   10

Does the child shout out whatever he feels like saying, whether it's in the backyard or in a theater? Does she grab what she wants wherever she is, perhaps hitting other children when they get in her way? Does he have great difficulty taking turns or waiting in line?

Problems with attention span:

1   2   3   4   5   6   7   8   9   10

Does the child spend less time than you'd expect watching, listening to, playing with, and otherwise reacting to what is going on around him or her? Is he easily distracted, unable to stick with things as long as others?

Problems with activity level:

1   2   3   4   5   6   7   8   9   10

Does the child fidget, flail about, run around, or otherwise move in ways that seem excessive or inappropriate for his or her age?

Social behavior problems:

1   2   3   4   5   6   7   8   9   10

Are possessions more important to the child than people? Does your son or daughter generally fail to make eye contact with others and to initiate play or conversation? Does the child show little concern for the effect he or she has on others?

Emotional problems and irritability:

1   2   3   4   5   6   7   8   9   10

Is your child skittish and oversensitive, withdrawing at the slightest noise or touch or at the sight of sudden movement or other visual stimulation? Does stimulation by people or things make the child cranky or tearful? Is the child regularly theatrical, impossible to console?

Problems with sleeping or eating:

1   2   3   4   5   6   7   8   9   10

Is your child a picky eater? As a baby, did the child develop colic easily? Does the child sleep irregularly? Did he or she sleep for only short periods as a baby?

Toilet training problems:

1   2   3   4   5   6   7   8   9   10

Was/is the child resistant to toilet training? Does the child have bedwetting or other elimination problems now?

A total score of 25 or higher indicates a significant problem with temperament. If your child's overall score on this scale is around this mark, it doesn't take much imagination to see that problems between the child and others are likely. Only a saint could fail to be aggravated by, say, a boy who does what he feels like when he feels like it, regardless of the setting or others' feelings; who may run around in a frenzy but overreact to the slightest bump or fright; who could at any meal refuse to eat at all and who believes that 1:00 A.M. is a perfectly suitable bedtime for a six-year-old. If you're this child's primary caregiver, you have a formidable job: You have to make a lot of requests of the child throughout the day, you're going to get a lot of *nos* in reply, and by bedtime you'll probably be very frustrated with each other.

Some of you may have circled all 8's, 9's, or 10's. If you're not just having a particularly bad day and feeling inclined to exaggerate, you may want to explore whether your child has attention-deficit/hyperactivity disorder (ADHD) by using the form on page 33. If you suspect ADHD is possible, you'll probably want to get a professional evaluation (see Chapter 3). If the preceding list doesn't even address most of the quirks you see in your child's personality, you may also want to seek professional help to rule out inherited predispositions toward other psychological or psychiatric disorders. First, though, fill out the Profile of Your Characteristics questionnaire on page 35, it may show that you're overreacting a bit.

Later chapters will go into more detail on how temperament shows up in behavior. For now, be aware that these traits will affect not only how your child acts but also how he or she thinks and feels. A child who has impulse control problems may seem selfish, bossy, and rude but really just doesn't stop to think about the consequences of what he or she desires right now. A child who has problems with attention span will want a lot more excitement and stimulation than the average child, and one with a high activity level will feel severely constrained by sitting still and being quiet. One who doesn't socialize as peers do won't be swayed by standard rules of conduct and won't appear to care much about how his or her actions affect others. An irritable or emotional child will get annoyed at the slightest obstacle, may treat a slight as if it's the end of the world, and may approach life with a glum attitude that seems unchildlike. What drives many defiant children I have known is the overriding desire to get what they want right here, right now. As you saw with Tim earlier in the chapter, many parents are puzzled by the fact that children know bedtime, mealtime, or homework is inevitable yet fight it day after day. Defiant children often don't look forward or backward in time the way others do. It doesn't matter that bedtime is inescapable; what matters is escaping it *in this particular moment.*

Body, Mind, and Maturity

Being "high-strung," "prickly," "difficult," or "demanding" can make your child defiant, disobedient, and downright rude in any and all individual situations. Unfortunately, other characteristics of your child can also lead, though a little more circuitously, to defiant behavior. Does your child have any intellectual or developmental delays? Is he or she suffering from health or chronic medical problems? Are there any physical disabilities? It's a sad fact that children are often mean, even cruel, when they first meet someone who is different in any way.

If your child is called names or mocked because he can't play the same games as others, has a speech impairment, or has a tendency to step on others' toes (literally and figuratively), it shouldn't be a surprise if the boy becomes prickly, defensive, or even hostile. On top of the negative reactions the child may get from peers is the disadvantage the child may be at if a disability makes him less able to understand adults' requests or how to comply with them and less able to control himself.

How about your child? Does your son or daughter have any such hurdles to overcome? List them and rate their severity below.

Health problems: _____

1   2   3   4   5   6   7   8   9   10

Physical problems: _____

1   2   3   4   5   6   7   8   9   10

Developmental delays: _____

1   2   3   4   5   6   7   8   9   10

COULD YOUR CHILD HAVE ADHD?

Over the last six months, which of the following behaviors has your child shown *often* compared to others of your child's age?

1. Fails to give close attention to details or makes careless mistakes in schoolwork.
2. Has difficulty sustaining attention in tasks or play activities.
3. Does not seem to listen when spoken to directly.
4. Does not follow through on instructions and fails to finish work.
5. Has difficulty organizing tasks and activities.
6. Avoids tasks (e.g., schoolwork, homework) that require mental effort.
7. Loses things necessary for tasks or activities.
8. Is easily distracted.
9. Is forgetful in daily activities.
10. Fidgets with hands or feet or squirms in seat.
11. Leaves seat in classroom or in other situations in which remaining seated is expected.
12. Runs about or climbs excessively in situations in which it is inappropriate.
13. Has difficulty playing or engaging in leisure activities quietly.
14. Is "on the go" or acts as if "driven by a motor."
15. Talks excessively.
16. Blurts out answers before questions have been completed.
17. Has difficulty awaiting turn.
18. Interrupts or intrudes on others.

If your child has six or more of the behaviors in 1–9 and/or six or more in 10–18, he or she may have ADHD and should probably be evaluated professionally (see Chapter 3). Save your answers for later comparison.

The Parents: The Old Block That Produced the Chip?

Dan's innocent question, "How was your day?" prompted this anguished reply from his wife, Sandy: "It was *awful*. Ben can't sit still long enough to do one homework assignment, let alone three. If he doesn't get the answers right away, he blames it on me and starts throwing his pencils around. He questions every little suggestion I make, like some sort of miniature devil's advocate. Then when he's finally finished, instead of taking pride in his accomplishment, he informs me that since it's my fault he has used up his outdoor time on homework, he won't have time to help with the dishes tonight." Exhausted from his own day, Dan could only snap, "Of course he acts like that—he's just like you."

The fact that this was probably the worst thing Dan could have said doesn't make it any less true. Sandy and Ben are very much alike in temperament, though they're at loggerheads so often that both would deny any similarity between them. Similar temperament is just one way that your own characteristics can contribute to defiance in your child. (And, by the way, notice that this chip-off-the-old-block likeness is, in turn, having a negative effect on Sandy and Dan's marital relationship, which, as we'll see, can boomerang back into exacerbating Ben's defiance.)

Like Mother, Like Son

If your child inherited a testy temperament or any of the other characteristics we just discussed, where do you think he got them? Chances are your child got them from you or your spouse. Let's assume, as is so often the case in my clinical experience, that you are the mother and primary caregiver and your son is the defiant child. If you do resemble each other, then your short fuse certainly could evoke defiant reactions in your short-fused son. Or your impulsiveness may lead you to speak or act with your child before you think, meaning your dealings with him could be impetuous, capricious, and inconsistent. Unpredictability has long been known to cause all young creatures—human and animal—lots of anxiety, which often brings out defiant reactions. Your similarities in temperament can take many other shapes, and the more severe your own problems, the more likely it is that they'll contribute to defiance in your child.

"Is That My Child?"

The reverse is also possible, of course—that you and your child are so different that you feel at a loss in managing the child. Where you're calm and deliberate, your child is excitable and impulsive. No matter how open-minded we are, we all have expectations for how people should think and act, especially our children. Behavior and attitudes that are extremely foreign are often intolerable to us, and we may overreact.

The Goodness of Fit

What this all adds up to is a quality you may have heard about elsewhere. It's called the "goodness of fit," and it means simply that you need to be aware of how your temperament dovetails with or diverges from your child's so you know where areas of conflict are likely to arise. On the following form, rate any problems of your own that you believe may contribute to difficulties you have in managing your child on the same scale as you used for your child earlier. If you're willing to risk making uncomfortable discoveries, consider having your spouse or another close relative fill out the form about you as well.

PROFILE OF YOUR CHARACTERISTICS

Health problems:

1   2   3   4   5   6   7   8   9   10

Physical problems:

1   2   3   4   5   6   7   8   9   10

Emotional problems:

1   2   3   4   5   6   7   8   9   10

Thinking problems:

1   2   3   4   5   6   7   8   9   10

Problems with attention span:

1   2   3   4   5   6   7   8   9   10

Problems with activity level:

1   2   3   4   5   6   7   8   9   10

Problems with impulse control:

1   2   3   4   5   6   7   8   9   10

Problems with moodiness:

1   2   3   4   5   6   7   8   9   10

Problems with eating:

1   2   3   4   5   6   7   8   9   10

Problems with sleeping:

1   2   3   4   5   6   7   8   9   10

"High" scores on any of these can make child rearing difficult, but it's even more revealing to compare these scores to the ones you got from your child's profile. Pay particular attention to problems you've identified in yourself with impulse control, attention span, and activity level. Many adults are now discovering, with the help of therapists, that they have ADHD. This condition is not only highly inheritable, which means your children may have it too, but it poses additional challenges to parenting. It's very difficult to be attentive and consistent with your children when you suffer from the problems associated with ADHD. You may want to get help for yourself before or while you try the strategies for helping your child in Part Two of this book.

The Parent–Child Relationship: Great Expectations

The way your dealings with your child tend to unfold is very much a product of the child's characteristics and yours, as I illustrate throughout this section. What you've learned about the two of you so far has probably already made certain typical clashes more understandable. If your child is highly active and oversensitive to touch, it's no wonder the three-year-old hates being bathed. If you have a volatile temper, is it any surprise that her resistance at bathtime sorely tempts you to spank her? This not-so-good fit can make any individual encounter a nasty confrontation, but does it have to sever the parent–child bond? Does it have to transform your child into someone who resists *everything* you request and spends her days fighting a series of hopeless battles?

No, it does not. Parent–child interactions cause defiance to grow only when they repeatedly follow the same negative pattern, teaching destructive lessons to both child and parent. In other words, it takes time. Here's how it goes:

1. By paying the wrong kind of attention, you unintentionally encourage your child's oppositional behavior. It's hard not to let your buttons get pushed when your child has a temper tantrum or aggressively disobeys. But although simply ignoring the problem doesn't work for most defiant children, neither does paying attention if your child's goal was in fact to interrupt what you were doing, get your undivided attention, or otherwise gain your notice. The trick, unfortunately, is to know what the child is looking for—and understanding that depends to an extent on knowing the child's temperament. Some children will act out to get your attention; others will act out because it puts off something unpleasant or gratifies some other strong desire, and ignoring them will be interpreted as tacit approval of their behavior. If you give the child what he or she wants or allow the child to evade what he or she doesn't want, you can expect a repeat of the defiant behavior in the future.

2. By taking an inconsistent approach to your child, you urge the child to seek predictability, even if that means behaving badly to get your negative reaction. When the rules change every day, it's only natural for a child to take a constant tack of testing parental authority through defiance. So, even though it may seem bizarre to you, if your son feels that he can elicit a predictably angry reaction from you by refusing to obey, he's quite likely to defy you on a regular basis.

How many of us can say we've never been guilty of occasionally rewarding the very same bad behavior that we usually punish? Imagine you're in a grocery store and little Suzy begs for a candy bar. Ordinarily you calmly and firmly say no, and if she throws a temper tantrum you quietly usher her out of the store and give her a time-out at home. When you follow this pattern consistently, Suzy learns that temper tantrums do not get her a candy bar. But if Suzy is already a "high-strung, demanding" child, and every once in a while you reply to her histrionics with "All right, all right, let's just not make a scene today," Suzy learns that *sometimes* a temper tantrum does get her a candy bar. With most children, that "sometimes" is plenty to encourage them to try the tantrum every time—just as gamblers are encouraged to slap their money down again and again by the periodic payoffs they get.

3. By showing that you have a breaking point, you ask for bad behavior to get worse. In situations like the candy bar scenario, the child learns not only that sometimes a temper tantrum works but also that a temper tantrum worked where wheedling did not. So the next time the child wants a candy bar she skips the "Please, please, *please*" approach altogether and goes straight to the tantrum. Ironically, this learning process works on parents as well. Over time both parents and child figure out that the more quickly they get enraged and threatening, the more quickly they get what they want—the parents get obedience or the child gets a reprieve from a command. When this process goes unchecked over many months, it can lead to confrontations that end in parents physically abusing their children or the children destroying property, attacking the parents, or even hurting themselves. This is how "No!" escalates into violence in some families.

As with everything we've discussed so far about cause, you can see that these three mechanisms often overlap and intertwine. Yielding to a tantrum but not to begging is a form of inconsistency in response. So is rewarding the negative with something positive. According to your child's mental records, your behavior simply doesn't add up. No surprise, then, that the child seems to react irrationally.

Now that you understand some of the mechanisms that encourage children to defy their parents, take a look at the interactions you have with your son or daughter.

What Happens When You Make a Request of Your Child?

Andy, age nine, and Tyrell, age eight, are a lot alike. Both are argumentative, rigid, and quick-tempered.

When Kay asks Andy to take out the garbage, his regular Tuesday-evening chore, he starts to grumble and whine. As his mother notices he's building himself up to a full outburst, she matter-of-factly gets up, turns off the Nintendo game, and explains that he'll be able to get back to it in 15 minutes as she gently leads him into the kitchen. As Andy collects the garbage, Kay smiles and thanks him, and when he finishes she kisses him on the cheek and tells him what a big help he is. He bounds down the hall to return to his game.

When Celia asks Tyrell to turn off the TV and come set the table for dinner, he answers, "Just a minute, Mom—the show's almost over." Without leaving the kitchen, Celia repeats her request three times, a little louder each time. Tyrell continues to ignore her. As her voice rises, he turns up the volume. Finally, Celia marches into the family room and says, "Young man, if you don't get into that kitchen and set the table this minute, there won't be any TV for you after dinner—or tomorrow!" Tyrell shouts back, "That's not fair," stands up, and starts kicking the base of the couch. "Stop that!" his mother scolds. "You're getting mud all over my new sofa!" "I don't care!" Tyrell shouts back. "You're not fair!" "Tyrell, get into that kitchen right now and set that table, or you're going to be in big trouble when your father gets home!" Tyrell turns back to the TV in time to see the credits rolling. "Now look what you've done! You made me miss it!" he yells, then he picks up the remote control and throws it at the wall, where it shatters. As he runs out of the room in a rage, Celia takes a deep breath and walks into the kitchen, where she starts to gather plates and silverware for the table.

What just happened in these two scenes is important to understanding defiance, but not as important as what happens the next time these requests come up. Andy realizes taking the garbage out doesn't take long and wins him points with Mom, so he does it without complaint. Tyrell skips all the arguments and goes right to breaking a candy dish the next time his mother asks him to set the table.

In each case, both mother and son learned something from the exchange, which they then applied to the next such situation. Andy learned that his mother wouldn't let him stall and that he got her approval for doing his chore. Kay learned that calm action and sincere appreciation got the results that she wanted from her son. If you talk to a psychologist, you may hear this type of learning called *positive reinforcement*. Tyrell learned that he could easily put his mother off and that if he wanted to get out of setting the table altogether a little violence would do the trick. Psychologists call that *negative reinforcement*. Here's how it might act on Celia: Tired of Tyrell's new destructive bent, Celia decides to "give him some of his own medicine." After he breaks her crystal candy dish one day, she runs to his room and breaks his beloved remote-control car. Tyrell ends up setting the table, and Celia concludes that requests and threats don't work—it's best to retaliate if she wants Tyrell to do anything.

In real life it's not so easy to recognize these mistakes or the lessons learned from such encounters, because the escalation of defiance—remember that slow but devastating glacier?—is so gradual. But look back and you're bound to recognize that confrontations with your child didn't explode into warfare as quickly in the past as they do today. Cause and effect can also be difficult to see when they're happening because they don't occur in an unbroken straight line. Tyrell doesn't have to get out of setting the table every day for him to keep trying extreme measures to evade the chore. Even occasional success, as with the gambler described earlier, reinforces the worthiness of his defiant strategy. If you could step back and review the pattern of your interactions with your defiant child over time, you would probably see that they often follow the sequence shown in the figure on page 41.

How Do You Get Your Child to Obey Your "No"?

Children will grab onto other slipups of yours as well. Let's say you have a three-year-old who's pulling groceries off the shelves as you walk down the aisles. Repeated orders to stop it have resulted in a little girl who is now throwing a full-blown tantrum in the frozen-food section, with a dozen pairs of haughty eyes surreptitiously looking down their noses at you, the incompetent parent. So you do the only

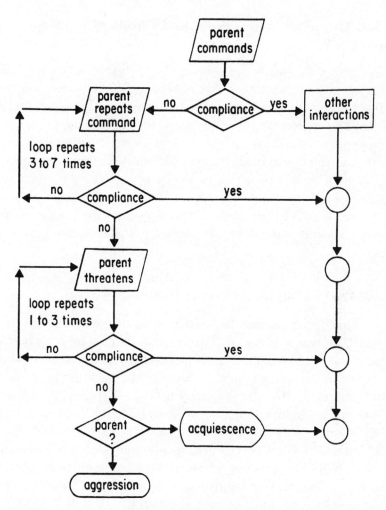

Typical sequence of interactions between parents and defiant children when a command is given. From *Hyperactive Children: A Handbook for Diagnosis and Treatment* by R. A. Barkley (New York: Guilford Press, p. 100). Copyright 1981 by The Guilford Press. Reprinted by permission.

thing you can think of: You pick the child up, walk over to the ice cream cabinet, grab an ice cream bar, and shove it into your child's grubby little hand with an "Mmm, this ice cream looks good, doesn't it, honey? Why don't you eat it right now?" Guess what's in store for you on future trips to the grocery store?

What Happens When the Child Wants Something from You?

Inconsistency also works against parent and child when it's the child who wants something. Say it's a school night, and your daughter wants to stay up an hour past her bedtime to watch a special Halloween TV program. You start out saying no, but she whines until she wears you down and you give in. A week later, she asks for a similar break, and you're surprised and annoyed when she keeps at you for a full 20 minutes and then refuses to kiss you good night when you won't give in. Why were you surprised? The week before, she successfully used negative behavior to get what psychologists call a *positive consequence*, and you can be sure she'll try it again—and again and again!

How Do You Reward Good Behavior?

Then there's your reaction to positive behavior from the child. Let's say that, for whatever reason, Tyrell obediently rises from his post in front of the TV the first time his mother asks him to set the table. As he walks by her on his way into the kitchen, she sarcastically remarks, "Well, *well*, since when did *you* decide to behave so nicely?" Tyrell gets no thanks, no approval, nothing positive from this encounter. How likely is it that he'll behave this way again? Or let's imagine that Celia is so stunned by Tyrell's obedience that she ignores it, afraid if she says a thing she'll "jinx" him and he'll start to act out again. Some parents find that if they make a big deal over noticing good behavior, their child seems so enamored of their attention that he'll do anything to keep it—including reverting to bad behavior—so they just leave it alone. Here, too, Tyrell gets no reinforcement for his good behavior and is unlikely to adopt it as a regular modus operandi.

Ignoring can, in fact, become an unfortunate way of life for parents of defiant children. They're afraid to acknowledge good behavior, and they've run out of resources to use with bad behavior, so they just start putting distance between themselves and their child's actions. The child, of course, usually takes ignoring as unspoken permission to continue oppositional behavior, and the defiance just gets worse. Because spending time with the child becomes less and less fun, the parents actually begin to avoid potentially rewarding shared activities. This is how the bond between parent and child begins to unravel. It is also how older children begin to develop serious forms of conduct disorder, involving covert criminal activity such as theft and vandalism, as well as overt acts such as physical aggression.

The parents' actions and reactions depicted in the preceding examples would not necessarily create a defiant child. We all make mistakes with our children—every day, in fact—and they don't have to be irrevocable. But combine a pattern of these mistakes with a child who has a difficult temperament and a parent whose fit with the child is awkward, and you have all the ingredients for a child with ODD. Now let's throw one more ingredient into the mix: the additional ongoing stresses that many families face.

The Child's Environment: How's the Rest of Your Life?

Other elements in your family's environment—the full catastrophe of life—can contribute to defiant behavior in your child as well. These elements include personal problems of the parents or other family members, health problems, financial trouble, marital relationships, employment problems, and relationships with relatives, friends, and other children in the family. Stress in any of these areas can adversely affect the parents in ways that contribute to defiance, they can affect the child directly, and they can have a reciprocal effect. Here are examples:

• *Marital relationships.* Research has shown that single mothers, especially those who are socially isolated, are most likely to have aggressive children. Single parents are often exhausted from carrying the extra burden of child rearing. They may also feel guilty about their separation or divorce and therefore are not as consistent as they should be in enforcing discipline with their kids. Single mothers also tend not to project quite the same authoritative image to their sons as fathers, and consequently the mothers may be tested more by their sons when no man lives in the home. Marital discord is another common problem. As I explained earlier, the parent—often the mother—who has primary care responsibility for the child naturally has to make the greater number of requests of the child and thus is in the greater position to evoke defiance. A smart child can pull parents' strings by setting them against each other, creating marital strife via defiance. Or, because of the difference in the amount of time spent with the child, the parents may simply disagree on the severity of the child's problem and the way to handle it. In addition, existing marital discord can put stress on the parents, making it more likely that they will be irritable toward a defiant child and treat the child with inconsistency, indiscriminacy, and inattention—which in turn will likely increase the defiant behavior, which could in its turn worsen the marital conflict.

• **Personal and health problems.** Stan keeps better control over his diabetes at some times than at others. When his blood sugar vacillates widely, so does his mood, and consequently his patience with his son Roy, who has been diagnosed as having ADHD and ODD. When Roy acts up, Stan drinks too much, which only makes his diabetes worse. And so the cycle continues.

• **Financial and occupational problems.** Maria is so worried about her family's financial future that she's taken a second job. That means 11-year-old Pilar is on her own until late in the evening, and her mother is exhausted and irritable when she is home. She snaps at her daughter, and her daughter snaps back. Pilar doesn't know how to handle the pressure of not being able to dress as nicely as the other girls at school, and lately she's started to complain of headaches, which only seem to make her temper shorter.

• **Relationships with others.** Gerry feels so alone. Despite having two brothers and two sisters in the area, all with families of their own, she has little companionship because get-togethers involving her daughter Lily are so trying for everyone. Her older daughter Julia resents the changes in her mother and her family life that Lily seems to have caused and spends as much time as possible at friends' houses. The 12-year-old's grades are plummeting, and in Gerry's last knock-down-drag-out with Lily the girl rendered her mother speechless by yelling, "You don't care what happens to me, and Julia already hates me!"

One more way that stresses inside and outside the family can affect defiance is that these stresses can simply cause parents to overreact to garden-variety childhood misbehavior. This may lead simply to parents consulting a professional and being reassured that nothing is wrong. But it could also lead parents to treat the child as if he or she is "sick" or "bad," which could lower the child's self-esteem and cause the child to misbehave defensively—meaning the parents' diagnosis becomes a self-fulfilling prophecy.

You may not be molding a monster from an innocent child, and you may not be in a position to change your lot in life. Still, if you're unaware of which parts of the child's environment are contributing to defiant behavior, you don't stand a chance of resolving the problems. Fill out the following form to identify the stressful factors in your child's life.

PROFILE OF FAMILY PROBLEMS

Describe problems that you perceive in each of the following areas, including how you believe they affect your child's behavior and your behavior toward your child.

1. Family health problems: _____

_____

_____

_____

2. Marital problems: _____

_____

_____

_____

3. Financial problems: _____

_____

_____

_____

4. Behavior problems with other children in the family: _____

_____

_____

_____

5. Occupational/employment problems: _____

_____

_____

_____

6. Problems with relatives/in-laws: _____

_____

_____

_____

7. Problems with friends: _____

_____

_____

_____

8. Other sources of stress (religion, conflict over recreational activities for the family, drug or alcohol abuse, etc.): _____**

_____

_____

_____

I hope by now you have a better understanding of what causes defiance in children and what may be causing your own child to behave that way. Sometimes the simple exercise of breaking down a complex situation into simpler parts and separately recording your observations about each helps you put together a more sensible whole. It's kind of like finding all the corners in a jigsaw puzzle and then grouping the pieces by color before trying to fit them all together.

I hope, too, that you now understand that much of the conflict between you and your child comes from characteristics that each of you will naturally find irritating to the other. Your child's temperament is not his fault any more than you're to blame for having a temperament of your own. Your goal in identifying as many potential causes of defiant behavior as you can is to recognize where conflict may be inevitable so that you can prepare to minimize it. It is also to change those contributing factors that you do in fact have power over—of which there are many. The next chapter will set you on the road to doing something about the problem with your new understanding of its cause.

RECAP: THE CAUSES

Although other problems or disorders—such as developmental delays and ADHD—may contribute to defiant behavior, in general four factors are involved in cause: (1) the child's temperament and other characteristics, (2) the type of interplay that has typically taken place between parent and child, (3) the parents' personality, and (4) the stresses of the family environment. Each factor affects the others, and in fact it is quite typical for the child's and parents' behavior to affect each other reciprocally, escalating individual conflicts and worsening the child's defiance and your relationship with your child over time.

Questionnaires in this chapter should help you identify major similarities and differences between you and your child—both of which can trigger painful clashes—to give you a handle on what makes each of you tick and how good the fit tends to be. If you haven't done so before, taking a good look at the family problems and other stressors in your child's life will flesh out your understanding of why your child may behave the way he or she does. Perhaps most important, though, because this is where you can exercise much control, is to become aware of how you may unintentionally encourage defiance by the way you interact with your child.

CHAPTER 3

What Should I Do about It?

Which of these statements most closely reflects the way you feel now that you know more about defiance?

> "I'm so relieved! I'm sure we can make some changes, and things will get better around here."
>
> "Now I'm *really* worried—our son seems to have a much bigger problem than the kids described so far."
>
> "I still have no idea what's causing *my* daughter's behavior and no idea what to do about it."
>
> "I feel awfully alone. How can I handle this complicated problem all by myself?"
>
> "Now I'm convinced there's *nothing* wrong with our son—it's all *us*. If we're the cause, how can we hope to come up with the solution?"

Where you go from here boils down to whether you now feel more confident and hopeful than when you opened this book. If you do, you can probably go on to the second half of this chapter to find out exactly how to use the information you've gathered so far to establish a plan for self-help using Part Two of this book. If, on the other hand, you have any doubts about your ability to address the problem on your own, don't hesitate to seek some of the help and guidance described in the first part of the chapter. Certainly, if you are now more concerned than ever that your child may have ADHD or another disorder that requires professional attention, make arrangements to have your child evaluated by a therapist. I'll cover the nuts and bolts of the process so you can embark on it prepared and informed.

Whatever help or support you seek, please share the program in this book. No matter what course of treatment a mental health professional recommends, the child management techniques described here can be adapted to enhance everyone's efforts on your child's behalf. If you should find—or start!—a parents' support group, sharing the principles laid out here may be a welcome contribution.

How Much Help Do J Need?

Identifying with any of the statements on page 48 except the first one is a sign that you may benefit from outside help. If you're now convinced that your child's defiance is severe, seek a qualified professional for an evaluation, diagnosis, and treatment recommendations. If you're still having difficulty sorting out all the possible causes of your child's problem, a professional evaluation will delve into the situation in more detail than you did in Chapter 2 and could guide you to a firmer conclusion, even if your child does not end up needing professional treatment. If you could hear yourself making either of the two last statements, various forms of assistance could be of benefit. Participating in a therapist-led individual or group parent training program may give you the ongoing reinforcement and confidence that you need. If you're generally a self-starter but in this situation you need a nudge forward, some sort of support group may be all you need. For suggestions for finding or starting one, see pages 58 and 227.

Those of you who are worried about a potentially severe problem won't want to waste any more time getting the help you need, so information on getting a professional evaluation follows first.

The Professional Evaluation

If your child is violent or, based on the questionnaire in the Appendix (page 225), may have conduct disorder, do not start on the program in Part Two of this book without prior professional guidance.

Consider getting a professional evaluation of your child if:

- You came up with a score of 30 or more on the Profile of Your Child's Temperament in Chapter 2 (page 29).
- You answered "often" or "very often" to six or more of the eight questions in the quiz at the beginning of Chapter 1.
- Your child is prone to violence.
- You sense a loss of self-control during negative encounters with your child or fear the child may be at risk for being abused.
- Your child fits the criteria for possible ADHD in Chapter 2 (page 33).

Consider getting a professional evaluation and/or consulting a family or marital therapist if:

- You came up with a score of 30 or more on the Profile of Your Characteristics in Chapter 2 (page 35).
- You have identified significant personal problems in the Profile of Family Problems in Chapter 2 (page 45), and you believe these problems are interfering strongly with your management of your child or with your own adjustment in any major life activity.

How to Find the Appropriate Professional

The person most likely to be familiar with defiant behavior and the methods for diagnosing ODD, CD, and other behavioral disorders is a child psychologist or psychiatrist. The best place to start, however, will probably be your child's pediatrician. Your child's physician will want to rule out physical causes before referring you elsewhere. This doctor is also most likely to know the qualified professionals in your area. Nevertheless, it's always a good idea to ask for referrals from several sources—your child's teacher or the school psychologist or guidance counselor, your family physician, any social worker with whom you've had contact, local chapters of mental health associations, or support groups in your area. When one name comes up repeatedly, that's the person to call for an appointment. If you get a varied list, try calling the offices of several to get a feel for the clinician's style and to gather preliminary information on the evaluation process; you may find it easy to identify the individuals you're interested in talking to further. If you, like so many of us these days, are enrolled in a managed-care insurance plan, you will have to follow the plan's requirements for such referrals. With any type of insurance program, be aware that benefits for mental health services may be pretty limited. Call ahead if you have any questions about your plan's coverage to avoid unpleasant surprises.

Don't underestimate the importance of finding a professional who inspires your trust and confidence and makes you feel comfortable. This fit is always an individual matter, but in general I've found that parents get the most help from therapists who have these characteristics:

• **They gently nudge parents into action.** Any therapist who immediately puts you on the defensive by being overly confrontational or appearing to blame you for all of your child's problems will only elicit your resistance to any treatment recommendations. At the opposite extreme, one who only presents you with dry, clinical facts may not provide the encouragement that parents in this often heartrending situation need to spur them into action. If you leave a professional's office after an initial visit feeling energized and empowered, you're in luck; if not, you might try another therapist.

• **They acknowledge your expertise.** Parents often come into my office so demoralized by their "failure" to raise their own child properly that I need to restore their self-confidence before I can help mobilize them. Remember, despite your recent conflicts, you *are* the expert on your child, and you already know a lot about child management. If you haven't been applying that knowledge consistently, it's doubtless because anger, frustration, and despair have thrown you off track. One of the greatest values a professional can offer is reminding you of the tools and the savvy you've merely put into temporary storage.

• **They speak in plain English.** Some professionals seem to believe that they aren't giving you your money's worth if they don't use all the 10-dollar words at their disposal. Others are afraid that speaking in plain English will be heard as talking down to you. The best therapists don't need jargon to get their points across. When nothing but technical terms will do, they define them or ask if there's anything you haven't understood.

• **They explain the reasons for the methods suggested.** How well do you think you could balance your checkbook if you knew how to add and subtract but didn't know which to use for a deposit or a withdrawal? I've found that parents who aren't told why they are using specific management methods—what concepts and principles underlie them—don't always use them appropriately and often don't stick with them long enough to make an impact on their child's behavior. Beware the therapist who only gives you a list of directives and then expects blind "obedience" from you. As the supervisor of this process, you have to be able to bend and shape the techniques a therapist gives you to make them work in your unique environment in the individual scenarios you encounter.

• **They empathize with your situation and acknowledge your accomplishments.** It takes effort to stick with the program presented in Part Two of this book or any other child management training program. The consistency stressed in Chapter 2 can be difficult to achieve without a little cheerleading, so look for a therapist who seems to understand the challenge you're facing, acknowledges the work you're doing, and reminds you that forward strides are largely to *your* credit, not the therapist's.

Obviously you won't necessarily know right away if you've found a therapist with all of these qualities, but the first appointment will usually reveal whether you've found someone who generally inspires your trust. As time goes on, a good therapist will always be receptive to your requests for clarification of information or modification in your working relationship.

How to Prepare for the Evaluation

At my clinic and many others, it is standard practice to send parents who have called for a consultation a packet of questionnaires to be filled out by parents and teachers. This gives the therapist a chance to review a lot of crucial information before the appointment and saves a lot of precious one-on-one time. Besides forms for recording your child's medical and developmental history, these questionnaires typically include behavior rating scales much like those presented in Chapters 1 and 2, but often more detailed. Parents may be asked to fill out a form that asks questions about the child's behavior in specific home situations, whereas teachers will be given a form aimed at school situations. When you fill out such forms, remember that the purpose of providing the information is to enable the therapist to make the best possible recommendation for improving your child's behavior. The therapist is not surreptitiously trying to evaluate you but needs to learn as much as possible about your home environment because it's so important to understanding the child's problems. Where feasible, many psychologists find it helpful to speak to the child's teacher(s), as well as having the school form filled out. You should not need to arrange for this conversation—the therapist will do so—but you will be asked to give your permission.

You can also help the evaluation proceed smoothly and quickly by taking time before your appointment to gather your thoughts. Sit down with a few sheets of paper and jot down a list of answers to the questions below. You've already recorded some of this information if you've filled out the forms in Chapters 1 and 2; consult those forms to save time if you like. Also try to be as candid as possible. Withholding information that embarrasses you will only handicap your therapist and compromise the accuracy of the evaluation.

1. What are your main concerns about your child's behavior? Divide your first sheet of paper into sections for home, school, community, and peers and briefly describe under each heading what specific behaviors alarm you—because they seem extreme or inappropriate for the child's age or for any other reason.

2. On another sheet, write down these headings: Health, Intelligence or Mental Development, Motor Development and Coordination, Problems with Senses, Academic Learning Abilities, Anxiety or Fears, Depression, Aggression toward Others, Hyperactivity, Poor Attention, and Antisocial Behavior. List any problems you see in each area. Don't worry about repeating items from your first page; reorganizing your thoughts into new categories can be of help in the evaluation process.

3. If possible, talk to your child's teacher(s) and make up a similar list of the concerns that have arisen at school.
4. For your last sheet, write the headings Personal Problems, Marital Problems, Financial Problems, Problems with Relatives, Job Problems, Sibling Problems, and Personal Health Problems. Under these headings, list all the family problems besides those of your child.

Save these sheets to take along to your appointment.

Finally, be prepared to supply the following upon request:

• Permission for the therapist to get reports from any previous evaluations of your child.
• Permission for the professional to contact your child's physician for information on your child's health.
• The results of your child's most recent educational evaluation (or arrange to have an evaluation done).
• Permission for the therapist to get information from any social service agencies involved with your child.

What to Expect at the Appointment

Always ask how much time you should allow for the appointment when you make it. Generally, though, the evaluation appointment will take two to four hours and will consist of a parent interview, a child interview, any testing of your child that seems warranted based on your preappointment questionnaires (such as an intelligence test, if one has not been administered in the last two or three years, to see if your child is developing normally in general mental abilities, or academic skills testing in any area such as reading, math, or spelling in which your child's achievement is delayed, suggesting a learning disability), and completion of some additional questionnaires.

The main purpose of the evaluation, of course, is to determine whether your child has ODD, CD, ADHD, and/or any other psychiatric disorders. But this is also where you begin to establish your relationship (and your child's relationship) with the therapist, with whom you may end up working for several months. Therefore it's important that you take the opportunity to express all the worries that have been building up in your mind. Don't hold back; set a precedent of open-ness and show the therapist that you welcome information and guid-ance. Don't forget to use the lists of concerns you compiled to remind you to get the answers you need.

If there are two parents in your child's life, it's important that both be present for the parent interview, since the two of you are likely to have different perspectives on the problem. Your other children probably won't be asked to attend. Whether your defiant child sits in on the parent interview will be up to both the therapist and the par-ents. Unless you are uncomfortable with the child's presence, a young child often can sit in on the interview. Older children typically stay in the waiting room, where toys are usually available for play.

During the interview, the therapist will cover all the areas already discussed in this book: your concerns about your child, what specific problems you observe at home and elsewhere, how each parent deals with the child, the family problems that may have an impact, and so forth. The therapist may gather this information by asking if various different situations are a problem, such as overall parent–child interac-tions, the child's play alone and with others, mealtimes, dressing, bathing, chores, homework, bedtime, TV watching, when visitors are in your home, when the child is left with a baby-sitter, and so forth. Whenever you indicate a problem, these more specific questions might be asked:

1. What does the child do in this situation that bothers you?
2. What is your response likely to be?
3. What will the child do in response to you?
4. If the problem continues, what will you do next?
5. What is usually the outcome of this situation?
6. How often do these problems occur in this situation?
7. How do you feel about these problems?
8. On a scale of 1 ("no problem") to 9 ("severe"), how severe is this problem for you?

By using this approach, the therapist fills in a picture of how you and your child interact and how the existing behavior problems affect both of you.

Whether the therapist interviews your child and to what extent will depend on the age and intelligence of the child. Whatever the child's age, it might help everyone relax about the process if you tell your child what to expect. Therapists usually ask children whether they know why they are at the office to begin with and how they view and feel about their own behavior. Other questions will be aimed at what the child likes to do (hobbies, sports, etc.), what the child would like to see changed at home or school, and how the child thinks other children view him or her. Some therapists will use "fill in the blank" sentences to elicit more candid answers.

Again depending on the child's maturity and mental abilities, the therapist will give more or less weight to what the child reveals in the office. Most children under the age of nine will not be too reliable in reporting on their own behavior. Nor should you be surprised if your child behaves differently (usually better) in the therapist's office than elsewhere. Therapists expect this and will not underestimate your child's problem because of those observations.

You may also be asked to fill in some questionnaires about your own state of mind, personal problems, and the like, probably while your child is being interviewed. Most therapists don't include these in the packet they send out ahead of the appointment for fear of offending parents. Your therapist will likely explain in the office that this information is needed to get a full picture of your child's environment, again not in some veiled attempt to evaluate you personally. Please be open to this process.

What the Therapist Might Find

To come up with a conclusion based on all the information gathered, your therapist will consult the American Psychiatric Association's *Diagnostic and Statistical Manual of Mental Disorders,* now in its fourth edition (DSM-IV). But these cut-and-dried criteria are rarely enough. The diagnosis of psychological/psychiatric disorders, especially behavioral problems, requires art as well as science. First, your therapist will need to take into account that the sources of information about your child are biased—after all, they're only human. Second, the therapist must tweak the standard diagnostic criteria here and there to adjust for weaknesses in the DSM guidelines:

1. If your child is under the age of four, his or her behavior should be more severe than the DSM criteria indicate to warrant a diagnosis of ODD. The APA developed its criteria for ODD using mainly 4- to 16-year-olds, and studies of large populations have shown that the frequency of ODD decreases with age. That means behavior that is severe enough to qualify as ODD in, say, a seven-year-old may not be severe enough to warrant a diagnosis in a two- or three-year-old.

2. If your child is a girl, she may have ODD even if her behavior ratings are lower than the standard required for diagnosis. The DSM criteria are based mainly on boys (a three-to-one ratio of boys to girls was used in DSM-IV field trials), and boys usually demonstrate a higher level of defiant behavior than girls. This means the cutoffs may be too high for girls. A girl who is noticeably impaired by her defiant behavior may qualify for a diagnosis of ODD even if she falls below the cutoff scores on the rating scales.

3. If your child is a preschooler—or possibly even an older child—and the defiant behavior has gone on for only six months, you and the therapist may want to wait a while before diagnosing ODD and treating the child accordingly. The DSM criteria call for a minimum of six months' duration of ODD behaviors, but two- to four-year-olds often act defiant for six months without necessarily having ODD. So do other children—up to 25% who are diagnosed with ODD don't fit the criteria a year later, according to some studies. Especially if the child is on the border for diagnosis, reevaluating six months down the road may be the wisest course. Labeling children prematurely *can* cause problems, as can treating a child unnecessarily. I don't advocate a do-nothing approach when the family is troubled enough to seek help for a behavior problem, but the program in Part Two of this book is a very benign form of intervention. Frankly, even if your child's problems prove short-lived, these child management techniques can only help.

Along with a diagnosis of your child's behavior problem, the evaluation should reveal whether your child has any other disorders, such as ADHD, bipolar disorder (manic depression), learning disabilities, or other problems. Identifying so-called comorbid (simultaneously occurring) disorders is important to the formulation of an effective treatment plan.

So is discovering the child's—and the family's—psychological strengths and weaknesses. Here's where all the information you supplied about you, your child's other parent, siblings, and other elements in the family environment is brought into play. Everyone's mental and emotional capabilities, ongoing stressors and sources of strength, and other factors will help determine what kind of treatment shows the most promise.

What might that treatment be? There are many possibilities. If, despite a child's defiance, the whole family is functioning fairly well, the therapist may provide simple parent counseling about ODD in a single individual session. At the other end of the continuum are children whose defiance and the impairment it causes warrants residential treatment. Most often a combination of interventions is the best approach. One example might be medical treatment or classroom behavioral interventions for ADHD, along with training in child management methods for the parents and social skills training for the child. If this sounds like an awful lot of treatment, remember how complicated the causes of defiance can be. Unless the problem is addressed in all of the settings in which it occurs—home, school, and the child's social arena—and unless all the factors that are causing it are involved, treatment is likely to fail. To make sure that you and your child meet the challenge, your therapist will recommend that you come back now and then for pep talks, reinforcement, and troubleshooting.

A Little Help from Friends

They may be total strangers when you start out, but the members of a group can be your most valuable allies while you're adopting the techniques in Part Two of this book and beyond. My colleagues and I teach the program in Part Two both individually and in groups. Whether we recommend group training depends largely on the parents' personality and preferences. Some people naturally benefit from the camaraderie and support of learning along with others; some, because they're shy, easily intimidated, or just lone rangers, do better one on one with the therapist. I believe the program is eminently usable as self-help, and that's why I've written this book. But there's no denying the several-heads-are-better-than-one benefit of sharing ideas and so-lutions with other parents. For an example, turn to Chapter 10. One couple's idea of having their child carry a picture of his time-out chair when they were in a public place where time-out on the spot wasn't feasible has worked for so many parents that I've incorporated it into this step in my parent training sessions.

If you do your best work and learn the most in a group, you might want to investigate finding a therapist-led parent training pro-gram. You can always use this book for reinforcement and reference. Contact a professional in your area—pediatrician, psychologist, psy-chiatrist, or school psychologist—for a referral. The availability of training will vary from location to location, so you will have to ask someone nearby.

Even if you don't feel the need for a training group, an informal support group could be of great value.Unfortunately, there is no net-work of such groups specifically aimed at parents of defiant children. Your best bet will probably be to contact the national office of Children with Attention Deficit Disorders (CHADD) (see Resources, page 227), since so many children have both ODD and ADHD simultaneously. Once you've found the closest local group, you can attend a meeting to see if it suits your needs. Otherwise, consider asking your pediatri-cian or other mental health professionals with whom you are working for ideas. You might even contact local hospitals or mental health clin-ics to see if a group exists or if there is a way to find out if there are enough interested parents to form one.

How much support you need may depend on the severity and na-ture of your problem, too. How aggressive is your child? Would you say he is more noncompliant than oppositional? That is, do your prob-lems center mainly on trying to get Johnny to stop ignoring you when you make a request such as "Please make your bed now"? Or are you trying to deal more often with Johnny's striking out, yelling and hit-ting when asked to do something he doesn't like, or acting hostile with no provocation at all? The latter behavior, obviously, is likely to be much more wearing on parents, and if you fit into that category you may be a good candidate for a group, where you can do a little venting and a little listening to others (who may have it even worse!). How about stress from other sources? If you're a single parent or one with marital problems, you're not getting valuable adult support at home and could benefit from a group. Likewise, if you have health, job, or financial problems, you're more susceptible to being worn down by your child's behavior—the empathy of others, as well as the clarity of their thinking, can help here, too.

If you do find or start a parents' group, share the principles from this program and whatever else you've found useful in this book. Be careful, though, not to give the impression that you are starting your own therapy group using this procedure. Only a qualified, licensed professional should lead such a group. In these pages I can't supply the ongoing exchange that a group provides, but I can offer a lot of the wisdom that the parents I've met have offered to me and to each other. Throughout Part Two you'll find inspiring examples of how real parents have used creativity and flexibility to apply the principles and techniques my colleagues and I teach.

Enlisting the Teacher's Aid

Don't forget your child's teacher when you're soliciting help for your child. As already discussed, your child's teacher(s) can provide an important perspective on the child's behavior problems at school. Don't forget, however, that the teacher may also have a unique view of the child's strengths. Many children surprise their parents by displaying talents and skills at school that never appear at home. When you talk to your child's teacher, be sure to ask about the positive as well as the negative. Also state your desire to help the teacher while you're asking for his or her help. Teachers today often have a formidable job, but the best of them will go that extra mile to see a child succeed when they know you're with them in the effort. Ask what you can do at home to help your son or daughter improve classroom behavior. The daily behavior report cards presented in Step 7 (Chapter 11) are a perfect example of cooperative home and school efforts that can have an astoundingly great reciprocal effect.

On a slightly more adversarial note, if you feel you're not getting what you and your child deserve from the child's school, know that you have federally legislated rights, especially if your child has ADHD. Children whose ADHD is severe enough to interfere with their school performance are entitled to formal special education services under the Other Health Impaired category of the Individuals with Disabilities in Education Act (1990). They also have legal rights under Section 504 of the Rehabilitation Act of 1973 or the more recent Americans with Disabilities Act (1990). For more details, contact your lawyer or consult the excellent text by Latham and Latham (see Suggested Reading section in Resources).

Your Essential Role as Parents

Now you know where you can get help in meeting the challenge of a child's defiant behavior. What can you do on your own? A first definitive step toward solving any problem is knowing what you can change and what you cannot. Temperament—your child's and your own—falls squarely into the category of "things you can't control." That does not, however, mean you simply ignore these factors in your child's defiant behavior. There is temperament—your child's impulsivity, your own rigidity—and then there is behavior stemming from temperament: your child's grabbing other kids' toys, your refusal to incorporate your child's motivations into the rules you make. Your job is to do your best always to make the distinction between your child's (and your own) inborn characteristics and the actions governed in part by those traits. Your job is to find ways to guide your child's behavior in a different direction without losing sight of what his instincts will tell him to do.

"When Kevin can't figure out his math homework at first glance," said his mother, Grace, "he skips the fuming and goes straight to an all-out eruption, throwing pencils, tearing up papers—once he grabbed his stapler in a rage and chucked it through the window, which was closed at the time. This just makes me see red immediately, and before I know what's happening I'm charging into his room threatening to take away all his privileges. Once I actually slapped him before I could stop myself. Now I know that we both have the same problem—we don't seem to have that little circuit breaker that stops people from overreacting to little frustrations. When I see Kevin turning beet red and flailing around his room over a simple math problem, I now see myself—and I also try to see how funny we both must look. I am the adult here, after all, and if I can't control myself, how can I expect him to? We're both working on it."

Kevin and Grace know not to waste time trying to become different people. Instead they're making an effort to understand how their temperament leads them down a slippery slope and how to put on the brakes when it does. That takes care of two of the major categories of cause in defiant behavior. What about the child's overall environment? Many people will say that there's nothing they can do about their life situation. They're stuck in a stressful or dead-end job; they married "for better or for worse"; they're not likely to wake up in the morning without the financial worries they had when they went to bed. Only you can decide whether any of the family problems you identified in Chapter 2 are in your power to change. Many will not be. Most of the families I have counseled have found, though, that the simple act of listing all the circumstances that may be affecting their child's behavior points to one or two that can be altered to some extent. Look back at your family-problems profile and do your best to find places where you might make some changes.

"Boy, I thought I was really on top of things when I changed how I reacted to Kev's homework tantrums," reports Grace. "He was suddenly like a little angel—at first. Then, the minute I thought he was ready to get back to work on his own, he'd throw another fit. Finally I realized something else had to be going on in his devious little brain. What made him throw another fit? Well, the fact that it happened the minute I went back to whatever I had been doing gave me a clue. Kevin really resents the time I'm putting in on my own homework now that I've gone back for my master's. And with his father constantly accusing me of being a bad mother, it's no wonder Kevin reacts that way. After going over a lot of ideas in my head, I came up with this solution, which seems to be helping: My neighbor babysits for Kevin after school while I do my assignments—Kevin's outside with his friends most of the time anyway—so I'm available to him at night. Ken isn't crazy about the cost. After all, I'm back in school so I can help improve our financial situation by getting a decent job once Kevin's a little older. But it's funny—now that I'm so sure I'm doing the right thing for my son, I'm not so sensitive to Ken's criticisms. I realize he's just awfully worried about money these days. So when he gets mad, I don't get so tense, and neither does Kevin."

I don't mean to oversimplify; this family didn't make lasting changes overnight. The point is that Grace approached her problem by looking at her son's (and her husband's) motivation, not just his actions, to figure out what could be changed and what could not. She also began to see how each family member's behavior bounced off everyone else's like a pinball and how she could use that property to start a solid winning streak instead of letting her family self-destruct.

What's missing from Grace's story is the nitty-gritty details of the changes this family made day by day, one small stride at a time, to improve Kevin's behavior in all aspects of his life. Homework wasn't his only problem, as I'm sure it's not your defiant child's only problem. Kevin was bossy with his friends, out of control at school, and impossible at bedtime, chore time, bath time . . . you get the picture. To reverse the downward spiral of worsening relationships that his behavior caused took concentrated effort from his parents. They had to establish a consistent set of responses to Kevin's defiance. They had to anticipate problems and be prepared to apply consequences quickly. They had to stop leaning so heavily on punishment and start relying on incentives for good behavior. When that good behavior showed up, they had to lavish it with attention. Because most of Kevin's problems were with his mother, it was Grace who had to spearhead these changes. Without Ken's support, however, progress would have been slow at best.

The habits of interaction that parents and children develop can be tough to break. The instinct to behave toward each other the way we've been trained to do is strong. That's why I've developed a series of clearly delineated steps to keep you on track. In the following chapters, you'll find a list of solid principles to lay down as the new foundation of your relationship with your child, followed by specific steps to take week by week to make the lasting changes that can restore the loving relationship you and your child both deserve.

Why is it all up to you when it's your child's behavior that's causing everyone grief? *Because the greatest potential for control of your child's behavior is in the child's environment, and an enormous part of your child's environment is you.* The one element that you have total control over is your own behavior. *That's why the program in Part Two centers on modifying the way you interact with your child.* Not because the way you act is the largest cause of your child's defiant behavior, but because it's the most amenable to change. You have the power to implement change, and I hope you'll use it, starting right now. Because defiance entrenched beyond puberty is hard to rattle, the child management program is designed for children aged 2 through 12.

Sam: A Success Story

Sam was a difficult child from day one. In fact, he had a lot more problems than the children of most of you probably have. I offer his story as an example of how the program in Part Two of this book may help even when a child has serious problems.

Colicky, temperamental, and difficult to console when upset, Sam proved stressful to care for from the first moment he was brought into his mother's hospital room following his birth. His parents, Lois and Richard, did not know what to make of Sam's mercurial temperament, fussiness, and irritability given that their first child, Susan, who was four years old when Sam was born, had always been a model child. A poor sleeper as an infant, Sam would wake at all hours of the night or day, rarely sleep for more than a few hours, and often fuss and cry when awake. Evaluated for colic by his pediatrician, Sam was placed on a soy milk formula in hopes of dealing with some of his irritability, but to little avail. There was little that Lois or Richard could do to calm Sam down consistently. Sometimes walking with him would suffice, other times taking him for rides in the car seemed to do the trick; but for the first year and a half of his life Sam's disposition and demands pretty much dominated the family.

When Sam began to walk, things got even worse. Into everything and a danger to himself as well as household objects, he required constant supervision. When frustrated, Sam often reacted vehemently, with anger and tears. He was quick to strike back at whatever resisted his efforts. "No" became his favorite response to his parents' directives. By four years of age, Sam was notorious with his neighbors and day-care play group. Bossy toward his peers, aggressive in his manner, demanding that others play his way or do as he wished, and total-

ly unconcerned with sharing or cooperating, Sam was quickly ostra-
cized by the other preschoolers, who avoided playing with him at all
costs.

Lois had Sam evaluated at a local mental health clinic, where Sam
was diagnosed as having ADHD and ODD. Because he was too young
for medication treatment, the family was instructed to read several
books on child management. But before they could start on a unified
approach to managing Sam, the parents separated, and Richard, a
schoolteacher, moved to an adjacent town. Upon their divorce, joint
custody was awarded, but Lois's apartment became the children's primary residence.

The divorce just seemed to make matters with Sam much worse.
He was becoming much more defiant, stubborn, and argumentative
with his mother and was becoming more physically aggressive toward his sister, occasionally striking her with toys when she was not
looking or hitting or kicking her when they had disputes in the home.

Meanwhile, Richard and Lois were becoming increasingly hostile
toward each other, getting into arguments in front of the children
nearly every time they exchanged the children for visitation. Harassing phone calls from Richard came in to Lois's apartment at all hours
of the day and night. Changing to an unlisted number did little good,
as somehow Richard discovered it, and the frequent calls, often with
no one on the line when Lois answered, were disrupting Lois's sleep at
night as well as daytime activities. Unemployed, Lois went on Aid to
Families with Dependent Children (welfare).

By the time Sam was five, Lois was being called to school nearly
weekly by Sam's kindergarten teacher over his unruly, aggressive, and
defiant behavior in the classroom. Sam was pushing other children for
little reason and hitting them on the playground whenever they did
something he did not like. Excluded from games organized by the
children, Sam would barge into them, disrupt the game, pick fights
with other children, or destroy what the kids had been making together, all of which further sealed his fate as an outcast. At one time, Sam
stabbed another child in the back with a pencil, resulting in his sus-
pension from school for a week, a hospital visit for a tetanus shot and
stitches for the other child, and the school's decision to hire an aide for
Sam's class just to help the teacher manage him and protect the other
children.

Sam's visitations with his father provided Lois a brief respite from his chronic need for management, supervision, and discipline. But within minutes of his return home, Sam was even more disruptive, defiant, and aggressive than usual, often for the first day or so following his return. Sam also began to insult his mother, saying when confronted that his father was saying these things about Lois as well. Sam confided that his father was advising him not to listen to his mother and that he should tell her he wanted to live with his father. It was easy to see why. On his visitations, Sam was treated like a king. During the few days they spent together, Richard lavished Sam with trips to the movies, new toys, dining out at Sam's favorite fast-food restaurant, and little if any restrictions on his behavior. There was no bedtime at Dad's house, he could take what he wanted to eat from the kitchen whenever he wanted, and his father would always take him out to play ball, go to the park, or out to the local shopping mall when he became bored. All the while, Sam was being told how stupid his mother was, that she was a bad mother, and that Sam ought to come live with him.

Life at home was becoming highly stressful for Lois. Talking and reasoning with Sam did little good. He would just repeat the same misbehavior, often within the same day. Lois tried to reward him for his good behavior but could not seem to do so very consistently. Increasingly depressed, she would withdraw to her bedroom, leaving the kids to watch television or entertain themselves, and would venture out only when the fighting between them occurred. Her periods of depression and withdrawal from Sam were occasionally punctuated with verbal outbursts and harsh physical disciplining of Sam.

Lois needed help quickly, both for herself and to learn to manage Sam, or she was likely to lose custody of the children to her exhusband. Her daughter Susan was spending increasing amounts of time at the homes of her friends to avoid the chaos and hostilities.

Things were falling apart, and Lois did not know what to do. She returned to the mental health clinic where Sam had been diagnosed, enrolled in a parent training class that taught her the methods set forth in this book, and also received some short-term psychotherapy for her depression. Sam was also now old enough to take medication for his ADHD, which greatly improved his hyperactive, impulsive, and distractible behavior. That, combined with Lois's learning how to be a more effective and competent manager of her son's behavior, began to set family life for them back on the right course.

Through her attorney she was able to arrange for the children to be exchanged at a neutral meeting place where a social worker would be present to minimize the hostilities that had come to characterize this now bimonthly event. She was also able to move into a duplex owned by her parents and next to their own townhouse, which provided her with less expensive rent, a chance for some baby-sitting and other help from her parents, and a new school for Sam, where he might get a fresh start with a new peer group. Lois also obtained a new unlisted number to cease the harassing phone calls from Richard. When Sam entered full-time schooling, Lois was able to get a part-time job as a dentist's receptionist, allowing her a chance to mingle with other adults, support herself and the children better, and improve her sense of self-esteem. Things were looking up for Lois and her family.

Before You Begin . . .

Sam's case was no fluke. The program in Part Two makes measurable improvements in children's defiant, oppositional, noncompliant behavior in up to 80% of the families who come through my clinic and in a much higher percentage among parents who are seriously committed to making change. I count you among that second number simply because you've taken the trouble to read this book. For the sake of your family's future, I hope you'll remain dedicated over the coming months. Here are a few factors that can make a difference to your success with the program:

1. Take a personal health inventory. Not much research has been done, but personal observations tell me that chronic health problems can hinder your effectiveness in making change in your child management style. It's common sense that running on only a couple of cylinders leaves you with little energy to make new efforts, so if you have nagging health issues that you're ignoring, now is the time to stop procrastinating and get medical attention.

2. How's your marriage? Defiant children usually have greater

problems with one parent (the dominant caregiver) than the other, and a marital rift can only widen this gap—to everyone's detriment. Furthermore, you'll need your spouse's support of your use of the child management techniques to ensure their effectiveness. If you and your spouse are having problems, can you take a first step toward healing the rift, if for no other reason than to cooperate in helping your child? Talk to your spouse, make the first move toward conciliation, try to warm things up in general, or consider counseling.

3. If you're a single parent, take a good look at your social support system. If the demands on you keep you isolated from your community, it's time to reach out. I know you don't have much time, but you'll be amazed at the new energy you'll have to devote to your child if you allow yourself the renewal of friendship and kinship. Are there neighbors you can reach out to, relatives you can invite over (or maybe ask to baby-sit), a support or social group you can join at your house of worship or civic center? These are not selfish pursuits; what helps you helps your child.

4. Don't ignore your own emotional or mental stresses. What may start out as garden-variety tension, malaise, or loneliness can turn into debilitating depression or anxiety. If you often feel anxious or depressed, get help for yourself so you can help your child.

5. Be realistic about your child's abilities. Children who have a mental or language age of at least two years can respond successfully to the techniques in Part Two, but no child should be rushed beyond his or her capacity. You're in a better position than anyone else to know when and how much your child comprehends. Let your child's understanding set the pace.

6. Be forewarned that many parents, after they've been through the program, tend to slip back into relying mainly on the punishment aspects of the program. It's an unfortunate fact that disruptive behavior is much more compelling than nondisruptive behavior, and when it demands attention it automatically elicits a controlling or punitive response from most adults. Whenever you notice a worsening of your child's behavior, review your own behavior. If you've been lapsing into overreliance on punishment, reread the principles in Chapter 4 to inspire you to accentuate the positive again. You can also keep a journal for a week or so, then analyze the information to see what might have gone wrong (details are in Chapter 12).

I can't emphasize the power of the positive too much. That's where lasting change lies, and that's where it all begins.

Before moving on to Chapter 4, take a little time to jot a list of your child's positive attributes. What do you like most about your son or daughter? What do others find attractive in your child? What does your child like best about himself or herself? (If you don't have a clue, ask!) Think back to accomplishments that made you proud of your child, events in which you felt especially close, moments when you laughed and played together. What made your child seem so special then? What positive characteristics do your child's teachers report to you? Sometimes teachers are in a position to see positives you haven't noticed. If all they report are negatives, ask them for the positives, too.

Now make a list of what the child likes—favorite treats, pursued activities, coveted experiences. Does your child have any hobbies? Is your daughter constantly begging you to stop for ice cream? Does your son save every nickel to buy CDs? Would your child rather be given a "gift certificate" to the bookstore or get a "pass" from you to the movie of his choice as a treat? Does she prefer solitary pursuits, like holing up with a new craft or model kit, or social events, like inviting a few friends to go bowling or rollerblading?

These lists are powerful tools. They remind you of what you can encourage in your child's behavior and what incentives you can offer for success. Even more, they keep you focused on the very special person lurking behind all that trying behavior, the boy or girl who wants your attention, deserves your approval, and repays all your care with matchless gifts.

RECAP: THE SOLUTIONS

With the understanding you amassed about your child and your family in Chapters 1 and 2, you are ready to make an informed decision about a course of action. If your child's problem is relatively severe, if you have identified multiple difficult contributing causes, or if you remain unsure about the extent of the problem, seek a professional evaluation.

(cont.)

Knowing what to expect will ease the process and ensure that you get the most from the experts you consult. Depending on your circumstances, the possibility of getting help for yourself, as well as your child, should not be discounted. Nor should you bypass opportunities to get assistance at school or from support groups even if you opt not to see a therapist. Wherever you look for assistance with this behavior problem, remember that you are your own greatest resource in learning to manage your child's defiance. Prepare yourself for the program in Part Two by taking care of yourself and reminding yourself of all that is positive in your child. The rest is just a matter of commitment to your child.

Chapter 4

Words to Live By: The Foundation of Better Behavior

When we understand how something works, a whole world of possibilities opens up. We can sum up our knowledge in laws, axioms, rules, and propositions and apply those laws to use, manipulate, and alter some aspect of our world. Without Newton's laws of motion, we might not be able to keep a car moving or send a rocket into space. Without Euclid's axioms of geometry, our buildings might fall down and our trains derail. Without the principles in this chapter, your chances of changing your child's behavior for the better are less than they could be.

You can accomplish a lot with defiant children by undertaking the program in Part Two right now. But you'd be missing an important preliminary, robbing yourself of a vital tool. Chapters 1–3 should have answered many of your questions about how your child came to behave this way and what you can do about it. This chapter synthesizes that information into principles that will reinforce your use of the program in Part Two and serve as the foundation for the future strategies you devise on your own to handle your child's behavior.

So think of this chapter as your fallback handbook. When you falter in consistent use of the child management techniques, it's your understanding of why you're using those techniques and what they accomplish that gets you back on track. Believe me, we all get lax, but that will happen less often if you remember what your underlying goals are. You'll find a summary of the principles on page 79. Photocopy that page and hang it where you'll see it every morning—perhaps on your bedroom closet door, inside your medicine cabinet door, or on the bathroom mirror—and throughout the day, such as on the refrigerator door. Go back to it whenever you feel you're losing your grasp of what you're doing and why.

The principles in the following pages are the fundamental rules for changing the life you lead with your child and in the process helping to ensure the child's happy and fruitful future. We've developed them to address the specific problems that exist in families of defiant children, but years of clinical experience have confirmed our suspicion that they underlie virtually all happy, healthy, productive parent–offspring relationships. In other words, these principles could be considered useful reminders for raising all children but are inviolable rules for parenting oppositional children.

A Fresh Start

Hopefully, you'll take heart as well as help from the following principles. They are, after all, predicated on the competence we know you possess. Adopt them and they can transform you from an indiscriminate parent into the type of parent you've always been capable of being.

Three New Ways to Think and Act

1. Know Your Priorities

When a child is defiant and oppositional, it's easy to lose your days in an endless series of battles. The more a child resists your authority, your wisdom, your requests, and your commands, the more important "winning" each argument becomes. Before you know it, you're demanding things from your child that don't really matter at all, just for the satisfaction of occasional compliance and conquest.

Right now I would not expect you to be able to stop in the middle of every heated struggle to ask yourself whether you're fighting over the important or the trivial. That ability will come with time and practice with the program in Part Two. I do suggest, however, that when you have a calm moment you sit down and make a list of your priorities for change in your child and in the relationship the two of you have. What's most important—improved school performance? Better behavior in public? Better social interaction with the kids in the neighborhood? Completion of necessary tasks like chores, grooming, and homework? A decrease in aggressiveness toward others? A recapture of warm moments between you and your child? If you aim your best efforts at your top priorities, initial successes in those areas will provide the greatest incentive for keeping up the good work. You'll also be teaching yourself not to sweat the small stuff.

Similarly, look at your own life. What takes precedence right now—career, homemaking, child care, care of aging parents, volunteer commitments, social life ... ? Be honest. A list based on guilt and *should*s won't serve anyone. Canceling the dinners out that give you respite and restore your sense of humor so you can "work on the problem with Joey" will backfire. Wallowing in guilt over your long workdays, which "must be why Shaundra acts the way she does," doesn't solve the problem. If you know your work is paramount—out of necessity or desire—you can look for practical solutions to the time crunch or at least devise a child management strategy that accepts this circumstance as unavoidable.

2. Act, Don't React

This is tough, I know. Parents of defiant children know all too well how difficult it can be to break out of the loop by which minor requests escalate into major confrontations. The techniques in Part Two will give you simple interventions to change that destructive pattern. For now, think *initiative* and *choice*. You are not actually at the mercy of your child. How you interact with your child in any individual encounter is your choice. The best way to take the initiative toward change is to have a plan for how *you* will act in the future. How your child acts will follow.

3. Act, Don't Yak

I quoted psychologist Sam Goldstein, PhD, for this valuable bit of advice in *Taking Charge of ADHD*. Carol, mother of ODD-diagnosed

Charlie, says, "The more I try to reason with him, the deeper he digs in his heels." Sound familiar? This is one of the most demoralizing consequences of defiance for many parents: The child's refusal to "listen to reason" destroys parents' confidence in their powers of logical persuasion. You can't be very smart if you can't get a seven-year-old to see things your way, can you? Of course, it has nothing to do with your intelligence (or the child's). It's just that defiant children (many of whom have ADHD) respond much more readily to an adult's prompt actions in imposing consequences than to talk. Charlie will shut off Carol's "undeniable" argument that all children have to get enough sleep, that it's too late to play basketball, that if he doesn't go to bed now she'll be angry. It's irrelevant to his immediate goal of postponing bedtime so he can keep shooting hoops. Her prompt move to turn off the light over the basketball hoop and tell him that he'll get five "reward points" (see Chapter 7) if he's ready for bed in five minutes gets him moving because he can't play in the dark and he finds the potential reward appealing.

Three New Ways to Relate

1. Try to See Things the Child's Way

It's hard to see anything but red when you're dealing with unrelenting resistance. Therefore, it helps to keep uppermost in mind that your child behaves the way he does because he really can't see things your way. Yes, Conner knows that baths are a fact of life. But his internal wiring tells him that continuing whatever he's doing for fun right now is paramount. His temperament makes him furious when you tell him he has to stop. His memories of having gotten away with this before urge him to keep trying. If you can remember what motivates him, you won't be as quick to hold his transgressions against him. A little understanding will go a long way toward easing the tension between you and getting you back on a mutually cooperative path.

By the way, seeing things the child's way does *not* mean giving in to him or her. It means keeping in mind that the child's perspective is very narrow, focused on the here-and-now of the situation and postponement of what the child does not like doing, while following through on your request.

2. Stop Blaming

As we've already discussed, it's easy to look for someone to blame for a child's defiant behavior. By now I hope you believe that it's not all your fault or your child's. But if you're holding fast to old guilt or blame, learn to practice forgiveness all around. I usually advise parents to spend a reflective moment at the end of each day forgiving their child for the day's conflicts and forgiving themselves for their inevitable mistakes and lapses. While they're at it, I add, they might as well let go of bitterness toward everyone else—the woman in the supermarket who glowered at little Beth, the teacher who questioned their ability as parents, the neighbor who won't let Jose play at her house. Resentment, stored hurt, and anger are poor uses of your emotional resources and make it very difficult to take advantage of the positive, rewarding events that come your way.

3. Keep Your Distance

I'm sure you've seen those cartoon fights in which a cat and dog dissolve into a swirling ball of dust and fur. You can't even recognize individual animals in the fray. It can happen to you and your child, too. After a while you're no longer distinct people but just one big fighting machine. Remember that you each can act autonomously; you don't have to react to buttons pushed by the other. Remembering your separateness also keeps you from beating yourself up over every little thing your child does. You are the child's parent, not the child's alter ego. Finally, a little physical and emotional space when needed can keep everyone cooler.

The Principles behind Better Behavior

The five principles that follow form the foundation of the seven steps in Part Two. Where Steps 1–7 make up a sequential program in which each step builds on the steps that came before, these principles apply anywhere, anytime. Because defiance is a behavioral problem, your management of it will always require you to respond to the way the child is acting. These principles should always be the cornerstone of how you treat an individual incident, how you encourage long-term good behavior, and how you minimize the inevitable misbehavior. They will serve you well in strategizing your own solutions and adapting everything you learn in this book to your own family.

1. Make the Consequences of Behavior— Good or Bad—Immediate

Unfortunately, one of the things that got you where you are today was inadvertently giving the child what he wanted most: to put off complying with your request. Whenever you repeat your commands four or five times before taking any action for the child's disobedience, the child has gained at least temporary ground. Remember, it doesn't really matter to the child that eventually she had to do what you wanted. Any time she gained reinforces in her head that her stalling or resisting tactics worked, even if only temporarily. (Maybe next time, she thinks, an even bigger tantrum will buy me even more time!) By extension, if the child has to repeat good behavior several times before it gets your notice, she won't waste her energy next time!

2. Make Consequences Specific

Children learn how to behave based on your feedback. If you react to Mike's punching his sister, failing to take the garbage out, and swearing at his father with, "You're a really bad boy!" he'll never understand exactly what drew your disapproval, and you can be sure he'll repeat all these misdeeds. Any broad response, in fact, to the whole child, the child's personal integrity ("How could you be so sneaky!?"), or the child's overall behavior ("Why do you always act so stupid?") will only confuse and demoralize your son or daughter. Remember, it is not the child who is undesirable but very specific forms of behavior.

The consequences of misbehavior also should reflect the seriousness of the "crime." If you take away an evening's TV privileges after your child steals something from a neighbor because you're in too good a mood to be "mean," the child will naturally conclude that stealing is about as serious an offense as failing to set the table. If you come home from a horrible day at work and ground the child for a month for forgetting to close the door on his way in, the child will be understandably perplexed. Finally, if you treat individual transgressions cumulatively, you'll only encourage the escalation of defiant interactions, as described in Chapter 2. Overreacting to your child's talking back right now because he's been talking back to you all week won't teach your child that there are specific consequences for specific types of misbehavior. Without this information, the child can't build a predictable framework of action and reaction to depend on.

3. Make Consequences Consistent

As you know from Chapter 2, lack of consistency may encourage defiant behavior more than any other factor. Unpredictable parenting makes all children uneasy, practically begging them to keep testing your limits to find out what the real rules are. Giving in or imposing meaningless consequences at certain times and in certain places actually trains the child to misbehave in those situations because the drive to get their own way is so strong in defiant children. I call the pattern of sporadic monitoring, conflicting styles between parents, and changing of rules from place to place and time to time *indiscriminate parenting*. I see it in a great majority of households with a defiant child. Establishing consistency in the management of your child's behavior is, granted, a lot of work, but it may be the single most important effort you make in your child's behalf.

We're all subject to our own moods as well as to varying circumstances, so it's not easy to enforce the same rules from moment to moment. The more you do so, however, the more clearly your child will understand what to expect following certain behavior. Grit your teeth and make 8:00 bedtime *every* school night, even if you're feeling particularly relaxed following a good day. Defiant children get so much negative feedback that one of the most important first steps (see Chapter 5) in improving behavior is paying attention to the positive as well as the negative. *Never* ignore the fact that without being asked your son has made his bed or that your daughter has put her breakfast dishes in the dishwasher—even if you're all rushing out the door to get to school and work on time. Children who get no appreciation for their positive efforts get discouraged and give them up quite quickly.

Almost all parents have trouble with consistency from place to place. It's pretty easy to give the child a time-out at home, but many adults are loath to draw attention to themselves and their child (and fear that the child will do something even worse!) in public or at other people's homes. Naturally, you don't want to humiliate your child in front of people whose opinion matters to him, but if you ever want to feel free to leave your home with your child, you simply have to make the child understand that he won't get away with behavior in public that is unacceptable at home. Chapters 10 and 11 offer lots of good suggestions for keeping the rules constant outside your own home.

Consistency between parents is a whole new ballgame and depends on minimal conflict between parents to begin with. Divorced parents may find it almost impossible to cooperate in child management, especially if their philosophies on the subject already differ. When that is the case, sharing this book sometimes helps. If not, or if the problem lies mainly in a relationship full of strife, marital or family counseling or other professional help may be the best route. However you get there, your child's future depends on a cooperative approach to managing the child's behavior.

4. Establish Incentive Programs before Punishment

This principle is so important that I tell parents they simply should call a halt to all punishment until they have been able to set up a specific program (see Chapter 7) for rewarding the positive behavior that they want to see replace the negative (such as brushing teeth versus refusing to brush). This may sound drastic and impractical until you take a good look at the typical interactions at your house. I bet that punishment has become the major (even the only) way you and your child interact. Further, I bet it's become less and less effective over time, because research and clinical observations have shown that without rewards for the positive, punishments for the negative lose their teeth. For both reasons, you need to start from scratch, supplanting punishment with incentives.

This principle becomes extremely important down the road. As explained in Chapter 3, once they've finished the seven-step program, many parents are sorely tempted to return to a punishment-only approach to misbehavior unless they hold this principle close to their hearts.

5. Anticipate and Plan for Misbehavior

When you have a child who misbehaves constantly, you can end up in full-time crisis management. Many parents of defiant children seem to be unable to plan ahead for these crises because there is so little time in between them. The funny thing is, though, if you were able to step back for just a minute you'd see that you'd free up a lot of time if you anticipated and planned ahead rather than handling each incident as it came up. Planning seems particularly important in situations where misbehavior can cause its greatest problems, perhaps inconveniencing many more people than just you and your child. I'm speaking of public places like stores and restaurants (Who has the time to cut holiday shopping short? Who wants to leave a restaurant in the middle of a meal?), but any situation in which you know your child is likely to misbehave deserves some forethought.

THE PRINCIPLES OF BETTER BEHAVIOR

Three New Ways to Think and Act

1. Know your priorities.
2. Act, don't react.
3. Act, don't yak.

Three New Ways to Relate

1. Try to see things the child's way.
2. Stop blaming.
3. Keep your distance.

The Principles behind Better Behavior

1. Make the consequences of behavior—good or bad—immediate.
2. Make consequences specific.
3. Make consequences consistent.
4. Establish incentive programs before punishment.
5. Anticipate and plan for misbehavior.

Learn from experience. Instead of simply dreading going shopping with your daughter, proactively plan, using first incentives and then (and only then) punishment, to set the stage for good behavior. Communicate with your child so that she knows what to expect, and you stand a good chance of minimizing misbehavior and its effects on others. See Chapters 10 and 12.

PART TWO

Getting Along with Your Defiant Child

The parent training program in this section was originated at the Oregon Health Sciences University by Dr. Constance Hanf in the 1960s. I am among the students of Dr. Hanf's who have gone on to amend and use this program in clinical practice, and I have made the most substantial expansions to it. Over more than 20 years, I've used the program to train thousands of parents and also introduced ten thousand professionals to it via seminars so that they could adopt it and train parents as well.

In my experience and the experience of my colleagues and associates, dedicated parents can make lasting improvements in their defiant child's behavior using the following eight steps. Mothers and fathers who have completed the program and made the lessons it teaches a permanent part of their child-rearing practices have many heartening stories to tell—stories of children with renewed confidence in their ability to get along with others and make their way in the world safely and happily, stories of close family relationships restored. I hope you will soon be able to add your own "happy ending" to this legacy. In fact, we would love to hear how you fared with the program—your triumphs and disappointments, the adaptations you made to suit your unique family, and any tricks or tactics you came up with that might help other parents. Sharing of ideas has been one of the cornerstones of our work with parents, so please add your voice to the ongoing chorus and write to us in care of the publisher.

How Much Time Will the Program Take?

Plan to spend about a week on each of the eight steps that make up this program. Please don't read Chapters 5–11 and then try to tackle all the steps at once. With any form of cognitive behavior change—and this program is a classic example—you need to give your brain time to register each benefit you gain before moving on. This "proof" gives you the momentum you need to keep going and to make changes that will last. (We probably all have several "crash" diets behind us to attest to the short life of revolutionary changes made abruptly.) Attacking the whole program in a rush will only force you to depend on quickly evaporating blind faith and rob you of crucial motivation.

Following the program in sequence is just as important as spending sufficient time on each step. Much research and clinical experience have gone into devising a plan that undoes some of the damage of the past while constructing a new template for future parent–child interaction. Specifically, we wanted to find a way to reverse the tendency to rely too heavily on punishment—one of the major problems we see in families with a defiant child. The best way to do that, we found, was to start with the positive, reminding parents how to use attention and incentives, and proceed to the negative (punishment) only after the positive was back in charge, where it belongs. Therefore, each step of the program is designed to build on the preceding ones, and following them out of order will only hurt your chances of getting as much as you can out of the program.

All told, you should see significant improvements after about four to six weeks of committed work. That's not much time when you consider how long it took your child to become defiant in the first place. Nor is it too great an investment when the return is enrichment of your relationship with your son or daughter.

How Much Jmprovement Can You Expect?

Exactly what will that enrichment look like in the real life led by your family? That depends on your dedication to the process, as well as the degree and nature of your child's problems. If you're diligent in learning the techniques in the order presented and you use the methods given throughout this book for avoiding "relapses," you can make lasting change, as 70 to 80% of the families we've counseled have done.

If your child is only mildly defiant or noncompliant and has no additional problems, you actually stand the chance of achieving a "cure." That is, your child can once again behave in ways considered normal and socially acceptable, and family life can return roughly to normal. All you may need to keep things on an even keel are consistent attention and praise paid to your child and the occasional use of time-out.

If your child has any of the more serious behavioral problems (ADHD, pervasive developmental disorders, or psychosis), hoping for a "cure" is probably unrealistic, but expecting noticeable improvement is not. Using the methods in this program, you can create an ongoing environment that allows your child to behave as well as he or she can. Like any prosthetic device, these techniques will help your child do what other kids can do, despite the child's behavioral limitations. Just as important, seeing the improvements that you've helped to make lessens your own distress over the child's behavior problems. It also inspires hope. You may even find that in time your child no longer needs this help. With long-term use, as the child matures and gains greater self-control, these techniques sometimes permanently reduce children's defiant behavior and thus eventually make themselves obsolete.

No matter how great the challenges your child starts out with, remember that the underlying goal of this program is not to "fix what's wrong" with the child but to improve the overall "fit" in your family. As you proceed through the eight steps, keep these objectives in the back of your mind:

1. Stay attuned to your own risk factors—those innate characteristics that you identified in Chapter 2 that may contribute to conflict with your child. Be prepared to change them where possible. Where that's not possible, think of ways you can prevent them from interfering with your effective management of your child. (*Example:* If your temper is as hot as your child's, learn to recognize when you've burned up your fuse and simply remove yourself from the child's presence until you can regain self-control.)

2. Remember your child's risk factors—also identified in Chapter 2—and take action to change any you can. Learn to accept and cope with those you cannot change. (*Example:* You can get professional help for the impulsivity associated with ADHD that often causes so much conflict between parent and child. Oversensitivity, on the other hand, may be hardwired into your child. If you accept it, you can smooth the road for the child by forewarning him or her of potentially disturbing imminent events, making change gently and gradually, and keeping overstimulation to a minimum.)

3. Remember the insights you gained in Chapter 2 into the way you set consequences for misbehavior. Stop using coercion, mixed messages, and negative reinforcement now that you know they only serve to create, maintain, or exacerbate defiant child behavior. (*Example:* Pay attention to what you say so you can catch any telltale phrases before they leap from your lips: "Why can't you clean your room like that *all* the time?" "Now you're *really* gonna get it!" "I don't care what I said yesterday. . . .")

Looking Ahead, Step by Step

Here's an overview of the program, from start to finish.

Step 1: Pay Attention!

Let's face it, when most interactions are battles, your child isn't going to place a high premium on getting your attention. Yet the "Look at me, Mom!" attitude that children are born with is a powerful incentive to cooperate. Deep down, even the most defiant of children really want your approval. So if you want them to do as you ask, your first job is to restore their belief that your approval is within their reach. In this step, you'll learn to balance the negative attention you give your child—from orders to criticisms to threats—with some simple, positive appreciation. The key is to take time every day just to be together—without giving commands, scolding, or correcting. Not surprisingly, most children enthusiastically meet their parents halfway in these efforts. Getting your undivided, uncritical attention for even 15 minutes a day can have an almost magical effect, rebuilding trust and compassion and mending fences right before your eyes.

Step 2: Get Peace and Cooperation with Praise

Now that your child is beginning to value your attention again, you can use that powerful tool to gain the child's compliance, as mothers and fathers, teachers, and other adults have been doing since time immemorial. In this step, you'll learn how to respond to your child's obedience and cooperation with acknowledgment, appreciation, and praise. Taking the trouble to say, "I really like how you made your bed this morning, Josh" increases the odds that Josh will make his bed again tomorrow. You'll also get in the habit of taking a break from activities you *don't* want interrupted—talking on the telephone, working in the kitchen, speaking to a visitor—to praise your child for playing independently and *not* interrupting you. This, too, will improve your child's behavior over time, increasing the periods during which you can pursue what you need to do without disruption.

Step 3: When Praise Js Not Enough, Offer Rewards

When defiance is very mild, praise and attention may be enough to win your child's renewed loyalty and cooperation. Most of you, however, will need more. In cases of ODD, the child's drive to get what he wants right now is exceedingly strong. Your job, then, is to make what you want from the child more attractive than what the child wants. As you know, it's often impractical to make your immediate objective (say doing homework) more appealing than your child's goal (continuing to play). This means you have to get a child whose focus is on the present to bank on the future. Vast experience in education, industry, and other realms tells us the way to do this is to offer future rewards for present compliance. In this step, you'll learn to use a variety of rewards and incentives to increase your child's compliance with commands, rules, chores, and codes of social conduct at home. Your child will earn credit toward purchases of certain rewards and privileges for obeying designated commands and rules. For 4- to 8-year-olds we'll use poker chips as tokens, and for 9- to 11-year-olds we'll use "points" recorded in a notebook. The child can redeem the earned credits daily, weekly, or over a longer term.

Step 4: Use Mild Discipline— Time-Out and More

Now that positive reinforcement methods are firmly in place and you've had plenty of opportunities to see how effective they are, you can begin to reintroduce mild forms of punishment. The first consequence you'll impose for bad behavior will be simply deducting points or tokens from the ones your child has earned for good behavior. Then you'll learn to use a highly effective form of discipline familiar to many parents. It's called *time-out*, and it's an old preschool standby for good reason: It's benign but very effective because it removes the child from what he or she wants to do by immediately isolating the child in a chair or a dull corner of the room. Because it's so easy to lapse back into overusing punishment, we'll take it very slowly at this step, using time-out only for one or two specific designated misdeeds.

Step 5: Use Time-Out with Other Misbehavior

Once you've become effective with time-out, you can expand its use to an additional misbehavior or two. This is a stage for refining the method, working out the kinks, and troubleshooting.

Step 6: Think Aloud and Think Ahead: What to Do in Public

Up to this point, you've been learning behavior-improving techniques in the relative safety of your own home. But it's forays into the wider world—stores, restaurants, houses of worship, and other public places—that strike fear in the hearts of even the most stoical parents. At this step, you'll learn to anticipate trouble and use slightly modified management techniques outside the home. Immediately before entering a public building, you'll establish a plan for managing misconduct, share the plan with your child, and then adhere to the plan while in the public place. As at home, you'll accentuate the positive by balancing any disciplinary measures with ways to keep the child busy during the event. Coming up with truly diverting activities gives you a chance to get creative and tap your child's positive attributes and interests. Many parents give their child's self-esteem a boost in the process by soliciting the child's help—"When we get into the store, can you help me find the Rice Krispies?" or "While we're on the highway, why don't you make sure I don't miss the exit for I-80?" or, for a younger child, "I brought crayons and paper so you can make a picture of our family for Grandma while we're in the restaurant." The "think aloud–think ahead" procedure works not only in public but also at home just before a major transition in household activities—when company is coming, when it's time to do homework, when a time-consuming chore needs to be done, or when bath time or bedtime is imminent.

Step 7: Help the Teacher Help Your Child

This step applies only to children of school age and requires the cooperation of your child's teacher(s). In our experience, teachers' willingness to collaborate depends on how much help they feel they need in managing your child's behavior in the classroom. By using a daily school report card filled out by the teacher, you can provide incentives—usually using the same token system you established in Step 3—at home to reinforce better child behavior in the classroom.

What's in Store in the Months (and Years) Ahead

Once you've invested a couple of months of effort into learning these seven steps, you should be seeing significant improvements in your child's behavior. (If you're not, you can take this as a sign that you may need more than self-help; go back to Chapter 3 for information on

getting professional assistance.) It's easy at this point to get overconfi-
dent or complacent, so Chapter 12 will give you an opportunity to anticipate what might lie ahead and how you'll handle new problems.
It's an old adage that as soon as you've mastered one challenge posed
by a child the kid comes up with a new one, and defiant children are
certainly no exception. Your child will grow and change, and you
would be wise to have an idea of how to use the procedures you've
learned for new behavior problems that arise. How would you design
a behavior change program for a second-grader who switches from
tantrums to hitting, a child who starts smoking cigarettes upon entering junior high, or a preteen who adds profanity to the disdain that
kids this age often have for their parents? I'll help you use your new
skills to prepare for such eventualities.

I'll also give you some ways to monitor and respond to progress
or regression. Some children, for example, will require the home token
system for years, while others will begin to accumulate lasting improvements that will allow you to fade this technique out. Chapter 12
will tell you how to distinguish between them and how to wean children from the techniques. You'll need self-monitoring, too, so this
chapter will help you spot relapses into the overpunishing mode that
is so counterproductive.

Features of Each Step

One step will be covered in each of Chapters 5–11. Each chapter includes several features designed to highlight important points and to
help you incorporate and adapt the techniques in the best way for
your own family. To give you an instant snapshot of how the methods
taught might look in your daily life, I begin with a couple of scenarios
illustrating how the lack of the technique encourages defiance and
how its use improves behavior. From there I enumerate the goals of
the step and reiterate how the step serves as a prerequisite to the next
step to help keep you on track. The meat of the chapter will, of course,
be clear instructions for what to do, with provisions for children of
various ages. Scattered throughout you'll find answers to common
questions and concerns to give you the benefit of other parents' experience, dos and don'ts, innovative applications devised by other par-

ents, and their insightful solutions to common obstacles encountered at that step. Helpful reminders of important points, as well as extra exercises and tips to help you get over some high hurdles, will appear throughout the chapters.

Homework Assignments 1 and 2

There are two homework assignments you need to complete before embarking on the program.

1. Take another look at the Family Problems Inventory you completed in Chapter 2. (If you haven't done so already, have your spouse fill one out now.) Now that you've read further, does either of you have anything to add? Do you have any new ideas for minimizing these stressors and their effect on your interactions with your child? I don't expect you to solve your problems over the next week, but you do need to formulate plans for reducing these stressors if you hope to get the greatest possible benefit from the program, so jot down a list of actions you plan to take. If you feel overwhelmed or helpless in the face of any major problem (marital conflict, health problems, substance abuse, etc.), now is the time to get the professional help you need. *Please don't launch into the program in hopes of changing your child without attending to your own personal and family problems first.*

2. Your second assignment is to childproof your home. Research indicates that oppositional children, especially those with ADHD, are more accident-prone, more likely to damage property and valuables, and more likely to create accidents for others than are normal children. Review each room in your home for potentially harmful agents or machines, for valuable property that could inadvertently be damaged by the young child, or for items that you wish to preserve or protect that are now within easy reach of your impulsive child.

Once you've completed these assignments, you're ready to begin.

CHAPTER 5

Step 1: Pay Attention!

Before . . .

"Come on, you guys," Nancy called to her three children as she looked up and leaned on her rake. "Let's keep it moving, or we'll never get this job done."

Jason and Dan, working together in one corner of the huge lawn, already had two big piles of leaves gathered and were tussling with the bags the leaves were supposed to go in. Their sister, Ellie, was standing on the other side of the lawn, her rake lying on the ground, twirling a large maple leaf in her hand as she watched the sunlight filter through it.

"OK, Mom," Dan yelled back to their mother, and he and his brother went back to their teamwork to rake the leaves into the bag.

Ellie seemed not to have heard her mother, who sighed. At least she's not keeping the boys from working anymore, she thought. Maybe I ought to just leave her out of it. Going back to her raking, she looked up when she heard Ellie shouting across the lawn, "Hey, you guys, come look at this leaf I found!"

"Ellie, I don't have time for your nonsense today!" her mother yelled. "Please, couldn't you just help out a little?"

Ellie picked up her rake for a minute but then dropped it when she spotted a caterpillar in the grass.

When Nancy looked up again and saw that her daughter still had not raked a single leaf, she stomped over and spat out, "OK, young lady, that's it. The rest of us have been out here working hard for an hour, and you haven't put in one second of effort. What makes you think you don't have to pitch in around here?"

Ellie looked into her hand and said, "Wow, look at the colors on this guy!"

Nancy grabbed Ellie's hand, flipping the caterpillar into the grass, and starting dragging her daughter back to the house, with Ellie protesting, "Hey, wait . . . come on, Mom . . . I promise I'll rake now. . . ."

Fuming as she returned to the lawn, Nancy began raking in a fury, mumbling, "I've had it with that girl. Well, maybe she'll think twice about goofing off when she realizes she's not getting any cake."

Later, Nancy relented and sent Jason up to Nancy's room to bring her daughter down to share in the treat, but her daughter refused to make an appearance.

"I'm not coming down!" she shouted as she gave her brother a hard shove toward the door. "She probably just wants to yell at me some more anyway."

After . . .

Nancy leaned on her rake, looked over at her middle child, and sighed. For every step forward they'd taken in the yard work that afternoon, Ellie had set them back a step—jumping in the leaves, running around her brothers and taunting them, refusing to do anything her mother asked. Now that they were almost finished, Ellie was busily pulling out the biggest, reddest maple leaves from the little pile she'd finally raked up. Nancy was just about to snap at her for the 30th time that day when she stopped herself long enough to notice the intense look of concentration on her daughter's face. Taking a deep breath, she walked over to her daughter and said mildly, "Those are beautiful leaves, Ellie. Maybe we should use them to decorate the table later. I've got something special in mind for tonight."

An hour later Nancy came downstairs after her shower and headed for the kitchen to start on dinner and frost the cake she'd baked earlier. When she passed by the dining room, the sight she caught through the doorway made her do a double take: Not only were Ellie's leaves arranged artfully in a crimson centerpiece, but the entire table had been set for dinner.

Like all kids, Ellie started out willing to do almost anything for a smile, an approving nod, or a "Good girl!" from her mother. But the Ellie in scenario one has gradually learned that her mother's attention is always negative—critical, demanding, disapproving—so naturally she's no longer motivated to work for it. Her behavior is getting worse, she's spending more and more time in her room, and fun family activities are getting fewer and farther between. An indispensable parent–child bond is beginning to disintegrate.

The Ellie in scenario two—the one we might see after her parents have gone through Step 1 of this program—hasn't changed her stripes: She's still obstinate and temperamental, quick to get distracted and to resist requests from her mother. But the downward spiral of misbehavior and family conflict has halted. Nancy is trying hard to appreciate her daughter's assets—such as her artistic eye for color and form— and to spend a little relaxing time with Ellie every day. Funny, the more time they spend in situations that don't require Nancy's direction or critique, the more of those positive attributes Nancy notices in Ellie. The more she acknowledges them to her daughter, the harder Ellie tries to please her mother. If they keep this up, the spiral just might reverse.

Over time, some parents stop paying attention to their defiant children altogether. Most, however, simply plod on, paying the wrong *kind* of attention: They ignore the child's positive behavior (or pay the child backhanded compliments for it), and they unwittingly encourage negative behavior by pushing the child's emotional buttons, by letting their own temperament rule their reactions, and by confusing the child with inconsistent responses.

From a distance, it's easy to see that a boy who believes he can't earn your smile by behaving well isn't going to try very hard to fight his defiant instincts. But you don't have the benefit of that distance. So your own instincts may very well tell you that if you correct him often enough, chastise him loudly enough, punish him severely enough, you'll eventually get through. It doesn't work that way, but parents get so stuck in this pattern that they blind themselves to what is happening: Consistently negative attention not only fails to "straighten out" your child but can do a great deal of damage.

Psychologists call their ideas about the parent–child relationship "attachment theory" for good reason. From birth your child is des-tined to count on you over all others for approval, appreciation, and acceptance. *Your* smiles and nods tell your infant that learning to stand up and walk is important—even worth the risk of falling. *Your* excla-mations that your toddler draws well or throws a ball straight tell her that she's a person who deserves love. *Your* patience, forgiveness, and understanding tell your son that he *is* loved even when he behaves badly.

When your child stops valuing your attention, you lose a lot more than a powerful tool for gaining the child's cooperation. You lose the child's trust, you weaken an irreplaceable bond, and you sacrifice a portion of your potential for guiding the child to a happy and healthy adulthood.

That's why it's so important to relearn to pay your child the right kind of attention, which is the goal of this chapter. The crux of this first step is a relatively simple technique called "special time" that offers deceptively complex benefits:

1. It will give you firsthand proof that the way you react to your child strongly influences how motivated your child is to do what you ask, whether it's making a bed or refraining from hit-ting other children.
2. It will teach you to notice and acknowledge good behavior and ignore bad behavior—rather than the other way around.
3. It will help you appreciate your child and the time you spend together.
4. It will begin to heal the wounds of constant conflict, restore trust, and rebuild the desire to help each other.

You won't reap these benefits, of course, if you make only a half-hearted attempt to learn this step. Because it sounds so simple, many parents mistakenly assume that learning to pay positive attention is easy. It's not. When you've been trapped in a vortex of battles with a defiant child, you have a lot of habits to undo. Taking this step very se-riously is the only way to gain the benefits listed above, and gaining the benefits listed above is the only way to make the next step effec-tive. In Step 2, you'll learn how to use praise to get cooperation, a measure that just won't work if your cheers are always punctuated by boos.

"But J Already Pay Plenty of Attention . . . "

Of course you do, but is it the kind that persuades your child to do what you want? If you're not convinced that the kind of attention you're paying your child is actually encouraging him or her to defy you, do the following exercise.

What Kind of "Boss" Are You?

1. Divide a sheet of paper into two columns and write "Worst Supervisor" at the top of one column. Under that heading, record five characteristics of the worst supervisor you've ever had. How did that boss treat you?
2. Now recall the way you worked for your worst supervisor. En-

---

Here are some of the characteristic behaviors that people remember about their best and worst supervisors. How do they compare to your lists?

Worst Supervisor	Best Supervisor
Makes unreasonable demands	Keeps things challenging but fair
Keeps changing his mind	Sticks to the plan; keeps us informed
Never says "Thanks" or "Good job"	Rewards successes large and small
Humiliates me in front of others	Shows respect and compassion
Blames me for her mistakes	Takes responsibility as the boss

thusiastically or grudgingly? Hard or as little as possible? With compassion and loyalty or with resentment and subterfuge?

3. Now write "Best Supervisor" at the top of the other column on your sheet of paper and repeat steps 1 and 2 for the best boss you can remember having had.

4. Take a close look at both lists now and ask yourself which column most closely resembles the way you treat your child. Be honest.

5. Finally, compare your own behavior under your worst supervisor to your child's behavior toward you. Is it possible that your child is merely on strike? Are you expecting him to labor under deplorable conditions?

Let's do something to change the environment.

Special Time with Your Child

To become your child's best possible "boss," make "special time"—15 to 20 minutes devoted exclusively to relaxing playtime with your child—a part of your day. Your goal is twofold: to learn to pay attention to the positives—your child's good behavior, achievements, talents, and other positive traits—and to regain your child's trust. The route to both, I've discovered, is to set up a scene that permits no commands, instructions, or probing questions from you. As radical as it may sound, I'm asking you to *let your child take charge.* It's only playtime, so it shouldn't be too hard to let him make his own choices and his own mistakes. Here's the hard part: Don't let a negative word pass your lips, no matter what's going on inside your head. Follow this plan:

1. Watch for a time during the day when your child is playing at something you know he or she enjoys, a time when you know you have 15 or 20 minutes to spare and nothing urgent or stressful to accomplish afterward. Without any fanfare, join the child, whether it means standing outside at the basketball hoop or sitting on the floor amid the action figures, and just start watching. Give yourself a couple of minutes to observe carefully and make a few mental notes. What is your child doing? How long has he been at it? Is this a continuing game or project picked up where the child left off a few days ago or a spontaneous new activity? Is there a goal, or is it just aimless fun? Is the child exhilarated or intensely absorbed? Planning or improvising? You may be tempted to ask the child to explain what's going on, but *resist the urge to ask any questions.* Disrupting the child's play even with simple queries may set the stage for the usual "Mom or Dad in charge" scene.

2. Now start commenting on what your child is doing. Keep your remarks simple and positive. Don't act gushy, forced, or phony. Just express honest interest in what your child is doing, punctuating your narration with genuine praise when you feel moved to do so. If your child is shooting baskets, you might break the ice with something as simple as "Nice shot!" and then progress to more specific details to show your genuine interest: "So, you're practicing your outside shot a lot. . . . You're getting better and better at rebounding. . . . I think it's great that you're working so hard at this. . . ." Or you can take a livelier "sportscaster" approach and actually do the "play-by-play": ". . . And he goes up for the layup—two points! Now he dribbles back and goes for the outside shot. . . ." Many parents, in fact, find that this broadcasting style works with all kinds of play.

3. After 15 or 20 minutes, tell your child how much you enjoyed playing together and say that you'd like to set up a "special time" to do the same thing every day.

In two-parent households (or in the parents' separate households), both of you need to schedule special times, preferably at least five days out of this first week. Special times should be a mainstay of your relationship right up to adolescence, though you can reduce the frequency to three or four days a week as time goes by. Don't be surprised if both you and your child enjoy these sessions so much that you'd rather hold them more often, not less.

During this first week, keep a simple journal of your experiences and observations during special times—what you two did together, how it seemed to go, and what changes you saw in your relationship, both during special times and during the rest of the day.

When Is the Best Time for Special Time?

For children under age nine, it's usually practical to set up a regularly scheduled time, whether it's when older siblings are at school or after school or dinner for a school-age child. Be sure it's a convenient time for both of you, a time when you're likely to be relaxed and able to focus all your attention on your child. If you're preoccupied by other obligations—such as starting or getting back to work or household chores—your attention will be divided and its effects diluted.

For children over age nine, you'll have to be a bit more flexible. Once they reach fourth grade or so, kids' schedules start to fill up, and you'll have to grab opportunities where you find them. When you see your child playing alone happily and you're relaxed yourself, just stop what you're doing and start an impromptu special time.

Do your best to find a time when siblings won't be around to compete for your attention. If that's not possible, perhaps Dad can occupy the other kids while Mom has special time with the defiant child, and then the two of you can switch.

What's the Best Type of Play?

The best type of play—no, the *only* type that's appropriate for special time—is *whatever the child chooses*. For kids under nine, when the scheduled time approaches, simply go up to your child and say (in your own, natural words), "It's now our special time to play together. What would you like to do?"

If you can do so without being bossy in any way, go ahead and join in, especially if your child invites you to do so. But still take a backseat and let the child pilot the activity. Otherwise, be content to be an amiable companion and an interested—even fascinated— bystander.

Defiant children are usually so used to being kept under tight rein that some *will* try to take advantage of this newfound freedom of choice. One clever six-year-old kept suggesting that he and his mother color on the walls. This, of course, was outrageous. But the mom outsmarted him by getting some butcher paper, taping it to the wall, and then proceeding to color the paper with her son. They even left their mural up for a few days for viewing. She told me she thought Saran Wrap might have worked as well.

One father had to trick his suspicious 12-year-old into special time by volunteering to drive her places as often as possible. Then, when the girl turned on the radio full-blast, Dad calmly made neutral comments about the music rather than complaining or demanding she turn it down. It didn't take long, he reported, before she was much more interested in spending occasional one-on-one time with him.

On a less successful note, one parent reported she didn't have much luck with special time because all her son ever wanted to do was play basketball and she hated basketball. Not surprisingly, this mother never did well with the program in general. Unless you're willing to relinquish control for this brief benign period, you'll have a hard time ridding yourself of your own bad behavior habits. If you can't bend enough to find a way to enjoy time spent with your child even when you don't favor the activity, you might benefit from a review of your own "risk factors" (see page 35).

Letting your child choose does not, however, mean going into special time mentally unprepared. You will probably find it easier to avoid commands and questions during some activities than others, and you should know which are likely to tempt you to take charge. Maybe you have a talent or skill you'd like to impart? An editor I know has to grit her teeth to avoid correcting her daughter's English when their special time involves writing a story. A graphic artist clenches his fists to keep from grabbing the paintbrush from his son and saying, "No, you do it *this* way."

I always advise parents that there's nothing they need to teach the child that can't wait until another time. Keeping that advice in mind may help you resist guiding or correcting your child during "dangerous" activities.

Other "hazards" may be harder to anticipate. To my surprise, I've heard parents say they couldn't help interfering simply because they wanted so badly to play, too. Before you interject, "Hey, it's *my* turn," remember who's in charge during special time. This is no time for rules. In fact, if your child has chosen a competitive game, let her invent new rules or even cheat if she wants to—without recriminations. Learning how to play a game properly is not a priority at these times. That said, cooperative games lend themselves to lessons in attention better than do competitive games.

As a final caveat, the only activity I would avoid for special time is TV watching. There's not much to observe but the TV, and "narrating" a TV show would annoy even the least touchy of children! Many kids instinctively choose TV, of course. We typically tell the parents to encourage the child to pick something else or just reschedule the special time for a time when the child's favorite programs are not on. A few parents have let the child pick TV and made this a snuggling time, with some talking involved, but I still believe the full benefit of attention is lost.

What's the Best Kind of Dialogue?

Rule #1: No Directions, No Corrections

No matter what else you say, don't instruct the child in what to do or try to change the way he or she is playing. This will only be interpreted as an attempt to take control, and the child will immediately fight the entire encounter. But if you narrate uncritically, your child will believe that you're interested in what he or she is doing. By extension, your son or daughter will come to trust your interest in him or her as a person all the time, no matter where you both are. The end result is a major boost in self-esteem and self-confidence.

One excellent reason for doing this narration, you'll notice, is that it keeps your vocal cords occupied, making it harder for you to disrupt the child's play with intrusive commands or questions. Believe me, when you've found it necessary to rein the child in 24 hours a day, questioning and commanding are very tough habits to break.

Happily, I've seen parents go to heroic lengths to avoid telling their children how to "do it better" during playtime, with excellent results. One 11-year-old boy chose cooking as the activity for their special time one day. That was just fine with Mom—until, that is, she had to watch in horrified silence while her son took an egg out of the refrigerator and put it in the microwave. Naturally, the egg exploded, and normally, the boy's mother admitted, she would have started shrieking at him. But because she was working very hard at "no directions, no corrections," she simply said calmly, "Look what happened to the egg! You know, I think I really learned something from this about heating things in the microwave—liquids inside solid containers seem to explode when they get hot. Very interesting!" Instead of getting defensive and denying responsibility for the mess, the boy amazed his mother by cleaning up the mess all by himself.

Rule #2: No Intrusive Questions

Here you have a tough balancing act. Children over age nine often find the running commentary form of narration stilted and condescending; with them you may have to ask more questions to convey genuine interest. Younger children, in contrast, recognize "testing" questions when they hear them, and they hear them a lot. A four-year-old will get her back up if you start asking leading questions like "And if we put these blocks together, how many do we have?" or "Which two colors could we put together to get purple paint?" These questions are meant to test children's development or knowledge, and children know it. For younger kids, try limiting your questions to the flattering, "I want to know all about you" cocktail-party variety: "Which block is your favorite?" "If we went to the art supply store tomorrow, what would you pick out to buy?" "How long have you known how to make this . . . ?" For older kids, just ask yourself these questions before asking any question out loud: Will my child have to stop what he's doing to answer this? Could this question possibly be interpreted as a direction or correction? ("Didn't you use a smaller piece last time you made this?" "Are you sure you want to color the White House chartreuse?")

Sometimes this takes quick thought and a careful tongue. One little girl, drawing a picture of her classroom, colored her teacher's hair purple. Her mother was stumped about how to react. She knew she shouldn't ask "Why did you color her hair purple?" (no questions). She also knew she should not say, "People don't have purple hair— they have brown or black or blonde hair" (no corrections) or "Don't color her hair purple; her hair is really brown" (no directions). She didn't want to say, "What beautiful purple hair," because she didn't feel that way, so she finally settled on describing the action broadcaster fashion: "I see you're coloring her hair purple." Her daughter was as thrilled by this description, she reported, as by the praise her mother gave her for other aspects of her drawing.

Rule #3: Praise Selectively

Here's another tricky balancing act. The goal of this step is to pay attention, not to lavish the child with hyperbolic—and therefore suspect—compliments. Praise, when you give it, should be quite specific. Although it's fine to say "Nice going!" sometimes, saying, "Wow, you have to have really steady hands to put that big piece on the little one without knocking everything down!" gets across exactly what you like about what the child is doing. You can praise the child not only for doing something acceptable—"I think it's great the way you clean up after yourself when you mix pancake batter"—but also for not doing something unacceptable: "It's great to see you being so much neater lately." Beware, however, the backhanded compliment: "I sure wish you had been this neat yesterday!"

When you do use general praise, be sure to have a wide repertoire. Kids are perceptive, and a stale spiel will invariably translate as lack of interest by you—the opposite of what you're going for. Likewise, a delay in praise will be read as forced, so always give your praise immediately following what inspired it.

Trouble Spots and Stumbling Blocks

"I don't need to figure out how to play with Jess. I just need to get him to do what I tell him to. Why should I waste my time on this step?"

Please go back to the exercise on page 95 and complete it now if you haven't already done so. Putting yourself in your child's shoes by remembering your worst boss should prove how important this step is. If you're really still not convinced, try a leap of faith, just this once. As I've explained, each step builds on the ones before, so, if for no other reason, complete this step because it will make Step 2 work for you—you need to improve the quality and value of your attending skills with your child before you can use that attention to increase your child's compliance with your commands.

I'm confident, in any event, that if you just hold special time for a week you'll see other worthwhile benefits. Special time helps to rebuild the parent–child relationship, which can only make your life easier and more pleasant. The fact that this is happening should be clear when your child, like most, asks you to extend special time beyond the usual 15 or 20 minutes.

HOW TO SAY "I APPROVE OF YOU!"
IN SO MANY WORDS (AND GESTURES)

Nonverbal	Verbal
Hug	"I like it when you. . . . "
Pat on the head or shoulder	"It's nice when you. . . . "
Affectionate rubbing of hair	"You sure are a big boy/girl for. . . . "
Placing arm around the child	"That was terrific the way
Smiling	you. . . . "
A light kiss	"Great job!"
Giving a "thumbs-up" sign	"Nice going!"
A wink	"Terrific!"
	"Super!"
	"Fantastic!"
	"My, you sure act grown up when you. . . . "
	"You know, six months ago you couldn't do that as well as you can now—you're really growing up fast!"
	"Beautiful!"
	"Wow!"
	"Wait until I tell your mom/dad how nice you. . . . "
	"What a nice thing to do. . . . "
	"You did that all by yourself —way to go!"
	"Just for behaving so well, you and I will. . . . "
	"I am very proud of you when you. . . . "
	"I always enjoy it when we . . . like this."

"Should I agree to extend special time? Is there a maximum amount of time that's effective per session?"

Generally, I don't encourage extending special time much beyond 20 minutes on a regular basis. It's too easy to push it to the point where things are bound to start falling apart. Both of you can probably hold it together easily for 20 minutes and thus gain growing confidence in your ability to get along. Of course, if you and your child really enjoy each other on occasion, there is no harm that I can see in letting things go on a little longer.

"I'm not so sure that showering my daughter with all this praise and appreciation is such a good idea. Won't she expect that kind of reaction every time she does the littlest thing that I expect her to do?"

The thousands of families who have undergone the program to date have not experienced this problem, so I don't think you need to worry about it. But really, would it be so unreasonable for your child to expect recognition and reinforcement for the efforts she makes? It's only what we all expect—from our employers, from our spouses, from the organizations to which we contribute volunteer time, from our older children and our friends for our love and care. At work we get that reinforcement via a paycheck, and we wouldn't be too likely to return to work if the paychecks stopped coming in. But even beyond that, as our worst-boss exercise showed, we all expect a little gratitude for our efforts. That's all your child wants, and it's not much to ask. Why not be prepared to give it? I can't think of a worthier habit to have, and I can think of many marriages that might be alive today if one spouse had not felt "taken for granted," which is merely another way of saying that his or her contributions to the marriage were unappreciated.

"I can barely get everything done as it is. I'm just too busy for this sort of downtime. Isn't there an alternative?"

While I sympathize with the time crunch that most of us feel today, I have to point out that assigning little time or importance to child rearing is symptomatic of many families in which children have behavior problems. If you're reading this book, you've already made the commitment to devote time to helping your child, so don't lose your patience now. *I can't stress the importance of this fundamental step strongly enough.* In my office I've suggested, only half in jest, that parents who can't find 15 minutes in their day for this worthy effort might as well give up their child for adoption.

Exercise your creativity here as elsewhere. I know one five-year-old who calls her special time "cuddle time" because the only time her parents could fit it into their busy schedules was before the girl went to bed.

"When I tried approaching my 10-year-old daughter while she was clipping pictures out of a teen magazine for her bulletin board, she immediately started grilling me about what I wanted. When I told her I just wanted to spend some time with her, she said, 'Yeah, right,' picked up her things, and walked away. How can I spend time with her if she won't even sit still?"

Begin the special playtime slowly at first, giving your child just a minute or two of your positive attention. Approach your daughter while she is doing something she enjoys, make a few positive observations about what she is doing, then leave. Gradually you should be able to linger longer each time, giving some observations and positive feedback as your child gets used to this type of attention. If this fails, take time to have a frank conversation with the child, saying you are aware that things have been very difficult and negative between you two for some time now and you really want to try to make it a better relationship. This is just your way of trying to do that. Most children will appreciate your candor and can see that you really do want to try to get along better with them.

"My five-year-old got really angry with me when I told him I wanted to set up a special time to play with him every day. 'No you don't! No you don't want to play with me!' he yelled before running out of the room. How can I ask him what he wants to play when he doesn't want to play with me at all?"

This can signify a very serious breakdown in the parent–child relationship, and you may have to face the possibility that you need professional assistance. First, though, be frank with the child about your motives. Say you really, really want to make this relationship better, and if you seem clumsy at first, you are sorry, but you need some advice from your son about how to do this better. Try a heartfelt, "What can I do so you know I love you and want to get along better with you?" Sincerity is often the key.

"I haven't had time to play alone with Robbie since Janie was born. The first time I tried sitting down with him, I was completely tongue-tied. The only thing that kept popping out were questions. What can I say to him?"

Just try describing your son's actions, but be sure to put a little enthusiasm into it. Some examples of how to rephrase questions as statements about your curiosity, interest, or wonder are listed below.

"In the middle of our special time Russell started testing me like he always does—talking back, mimicking me, getting a little physical—and I was having a really hard time keeping it together. What should I have done?"

When a child starts to misbehave during special time, simply turn away and look somewhere else for a minute. Often the immediate loss

---

TURNING QUESTIONS INTO STATEMENTS

Question	**Rephrased as . . .**
"What are you doing?"	"I don't think I understand what's happening here, but it sure looks interesting."
"Where did you learn that?"	"I've never seen you do that before now; I bet you learned that at school."
"Why would you do it that way?"	"My, what a clever way to do this."
"What color is that?"	"I don't think I have ever seen a color quite like that one before."
"How is this supposed to work?"	"You know, I'm really curious to to see how all this will work when it's done."

of your positive attention will be met with regret and your child will clean up his act. If he does, in fact, that's a sign that you're seeing the results you should be getting from attending positively to positive behavior and ignoring negative behavior. Don't expect to see this effect all at once, though. At first your child is likely to try all of his usual tricks, and you need to persist in responding with new tricks of your own.

One father was bothered by the way his son talked with his mouth full whenever he had his customary snack during their special time. His "new trick" was to praise the boy lavishly every time he said anything without food in his mouth and to stop talking and casually look away whenever his son talked with food in his mouth. The boy cut down on talking with his mouth full almost instantly.

"My son is no dummy, and he's obviously figured out he can work this 'no directions, no corrections' business to his advantage. The other day he started throwing food all over the kitchen and calling me foul names during our special time, and I just stood there without a clue about what to do. What should I do next time this happens?"

As you know, many defiant kids merely escalate their misbehavior when you ignore it because they know they'll eventually reach your breaking point. If turning away from a disruptive child doesn't do the trick, the best response is simply to say that the special time is over and you can start it again when the child is behaving better. Then get up and exit to leave no room for doubt. On the rare occasion that the child is so out of hand that punishment truly seems necessary, use whatever discipline you're accustomed to using and try again tomorrow. Later in the program you'll learn effective discipline to replace your current approach to punishment.

"My son and I have had special time every day for this entire week, and I really don't see any difference. He still gives me a hard time about every single thing. How do I know this is working—and worth pursuing?"

I would never promise that learning to pay positive attention to your child will change the child's innate tendency to be defiant—or that you'll gain peace and tranquillity at home overnight. Remember, you are doing this not so much to please your child at the moment as to practice the skills of a good supervisor—to try to be more observant of your child's actions and give positive feedback. If *you* are improving in these areas, the technique is working. As to your son's behavior, please be patient. It took years for things to get this way; they won't change overnight.

One thing I hear over and over from parents who have completed one week of special time is that parent and child seem to have gained a new perspective on each other. "For the first time in months my daughter isn't avoiding me like the plague," said one mother. "She actually seeks me out sometimes instead of coming home from school and running directly to her room without ever turning back! Yesterday I suddenly realized when we were talking in the kitchen that we were having an unscheduled 'special time'—no fights, no inquisitions, just a relaxing mother–daughter talk. And I learned more about what was going on in school in that 10 minutes than she'd told me all last semester."

What's happening, sometimes without conscious recognition by parent and child, is that each is beginning to find the other more desirable to be with. You're not just contriving interest in your child to get a certain response. Now your son or daughter is actually becoming more interesting, more admirable, more fun to be around. Special time is no longer an obligation but a privilege. The spiral is pointing up again. Let's keep it going that way.

"What should I do about Tonya's brother and sister, who may want this kind of time with me?"

This all depends on how old the siblings are. If they are close in age to Tonya, you should probably schedule a separate special time with them. If they are three or more years apart, it is not likely to be as much of a problem for the siblings. Even then, be sure to take some one-on-one time with each of them when opportunities to do so arise.

"Can I use this special playtime as a reward or incentive to get my child to listen to me?"

No! The special playtime is intended as a time for you to practice being a better supervisor, not to reward your child for things he or she has done for you earlier that day. Nor should you withhold special time just because your child may have misbehaved earlier that day. The purpose of special time is parental practice at supervision. The fact that most children enjoy it is just a positive by-product.

CHAPTER 6

Step 2: Start Earning Peace and Cooperation with Praise

Before . . .

Without looking up from the cutting board where she was chopping celery, Lee called, "Norm, why don't you start picking up those cars, OK? Your aunt and uncle will be here for dinner soon. We want the room to look good for company, don't we?"

The only sound coming from the family room was the blaring of the TV.

"Norm!" Lee's voice got louder. "Did you hear me? I want those toys picked up!"

No answer.

"Norman! If I have to ask you one more time, there won't be any Nintendo for a whole week!"

"Yeah, right," eight-year-old Norm muttered from the family room.

His mother poked her head out from the kitchen and said, "I mean it, Norm. Now."

Slowly Norm pulled himself up from the floor, one Matchbox car in hand. The minute his mother's head popped back out of sight, he plopped back to the carpet and started playing again.

This time his mother came all the way into the family room. "OK, Norm, start picking up those cars, and when you've finished that turn off the TV, then go get a dust cloth and wipe off the tables in here . . . and while you're at it, don't forget your own room. You still haven't made your bed." Lee stood by while Norm started picking up the cars again, then said, "Oh, no—look how late it is," and dashed back into the kitchen.

Ten minutes later: "How's it going, Norm?"

No answer.

Lee threw down her dish towel and stormed into the family room. Cars were still strewn everywhere and the TV was still blasting. In fact, every-thing was exactly as she'd left it except for one item: Her son was nowhere to be seen.

After . . .

Lee put down her knife and walked into the family room. Turning down the sound on the TV and standing in front of the screen, she said, "Norm, it's time to clean up." She waited until her son looked up at her and then added, "Please stop playing and put away your cars now."

Her son looked blankly at her, so she said, "Do you understand?"

"Yes," he said and picked up another car.

Lee stooped down, took the car from his hand, and gently tilted his chin up again so she was sure he could see her. "What do you need to do right now?"

Grudgingly, Norm mumbled, "Put away my cars."

"That's right," Lee said cheerfully, turning off the TV. "I'm going to set the timer for 10 minutes and do the dusting in here while you clean up the floor. If you finish putting away all your cars before the timer rings, you can play Nintendo for 15 minutes before we get started on something else."

Five minutes later, after some intermittent cheerleading—"You're doing a great job, Norm!" and "Boy, I didn't know you could hold that many cars at once!"—Lee and Norm finished their chores at the same time.

"Wow," said Lee, "you did such a great job—and so fast! Let's change that 15 minutes of Nintendo to 20!"

In scenario two Lee does everything right to get her son to do what she wants when she wants it: She cuts out distractions, then makes a simple command, asks Norm to do only one thing at a time, and makes sure he's listening and understands. Lee offers an incentive for compliance, sets a time limit for the task, and then stays in the room to monitor and offer praise to keep Norm going. Finally, and perhaps most important of all, she gives him kudos for his success and an extra reward for going above and beyond what she asked. Norm may not become a paragon of cooperation overnight, but as Lee keeps this up, Norm's motivation to comply will increase.

You might see scenario one unfold in homes across America any day, and it wouldn't necessarily be a sign of trouble. Asking rather than stating a command, threatening punishment rather than offering incentives, and making a string of requests at once may work just fine for some kids or on some occasions. But when a child, like Norm, already has risk factors for defiance, this approach, especially failing to monitor the child and praise him for compliance, can and will turn a potential behavior problem into a raging actual one.

In Step 1, you learned to pay positive attention to your child's positive behavior within the setting of playtime. Lee reports that even though the practice of special times hasn't made Norm any more obedient than he ever was, at least scenario one "didn't turn into the usual ugly screaming match." To get Norm to start complying with her wishes, Lee has to start applying her new attention skills to "work" as well as play. As we saw in scenario one, she didn't pay much attention to Norm when she told him to clean up (Did he hear her and understand?), she didn't keep an eye on him during the chore (*Was* he cleaning up?), and she didn't follow through (Did he finish the job?). Nor did she acknowledge and praise him along the way. Norm responded in kind: He paid no attention.

Step 2 is all about using your now-valuable attention and praise to get to scenario two and beyond—to get your child to do what you ask and to leave you alone when you need to get something done. The entire step is predicated on the fact that your attention *is* taking on renewed value with your child, so make sure you've succeeded in learning to pay positive attention via Step 1:

- Review the "special times" journal you kept. Did you report any improvement in how consistently and easily you were able to pay attention while sticking to the "no directions, no corrections" rule? The important thing is that your child received the attention, even if he or she did not acknowledge it. If you believe your attention skills improved over the week, they probably did.
- If you're in doubt, check what you logged about your child's

special-time behavior over the week: Were there fewer disruptions toward the end of the week than at the beginning? Did your child begin to drop any suspicions about your motives for planning special times together? These are certainly signs that your child noticed your attention and thus began to value it again.

• Did anything change outside of special times? Did your child begin to seek you out? Were you getting a few more hugs than scowls? One of the most immediate benefits of positive attention is the rebuilding of a trusting, close relationship. Remember, what goes around comes around.

• Sometimes the best measure of whether you successfully completed Step 1 is how *you* feel. Remember, your child's acknowledgment of your attention is not crucial at this stage. What matters is that you began to learn to see the positive in your child. A sure sign of that is increased delight in your son or daughter—noticing the admirable traits, learning surprising new things about him or her, wanting to spend more time together.

I hope you're ready to move on. Remember to continue to hold special times three or four times a week. Here's what you'll need to do in Step 2:

1. Work on increasing your child's compliance using three main techniques:
   a. Pay attention and give praise whenever your child complies with any request.
   b. Set up very short "training sessions" in which you give a quick series of extremely simple, benign commands ("Please hand me that pencil") to get your child used to how easy it is to comply.
   c. Learn to give more effective commands. (Here's a chance to apply your attention skills to yourself!)
2. Encourage your child to be less disruptive when you need to get something done by offering attention and praise when the child resists interrupting.
3. Keep defiance from disrupting the rest of your child's life by making a point of checking on him around your home and in the neigborhood.

Increasing Compliance

Catch Your Child Being Good

From Step 1 you know how much your child enjoys your attention and praise during playtime. Now is your chance to see the effect of this positive consequence on compliance. The key to this technique is to be quick; your attention will sink in most deeply when you respond *immediately*. The first thing you'll learn this week is to pay scrupulous attention every single time your child does what you ask.

1. This week, whenever you give a command to your child—whether it's "Brush your teeth," "Do your homework," or "Stop pulling the dog's tail"—instead of walking away to attend to your own business, as most of us usually do, stay with the child and watch.

2. If the child disobeys, handle the situation just as you ordinarily would. Don't try to come up with new methods of discipline. If the child begins to obey, immediately acknowledge it: "I like it when you do as I ask," "Look at how well you're . . . ," and "Thanks for . . ." are just a few examples of what you can say to use positive attention to reinforce the child's compliance.

3. If you absolutely must, you can leave the room briefly, but be sure to return regularly while the task is being done. Keep heaping on the praise as long as your child is doing what you asked.

• *Follow these instructions for virtually every command you give this week.*

• *Notice which commands your child follows inconsistently, choose two or three of those, and make a special effort over the next week to praise the child for fulfilling these particular requests.*

• *Add a small reward—a little toy, favorite snack, or extra privilege—to the praise when you catch your child being good without being asked.* Even defiant children may do the right thing on their own sometimes. One father was amazed to see his five-year-old son, who had been told what a great job he did in helping with the laundry, put *everyone's* laundry away for the rest of the week. Following a household rule *without* being reminded or doing an assigned chore without a parental order is exactly what you're after. It's essential, then, that you not let these achievements slip by unnoticed. Look sharp!

Show How Easy Cooperation Is

Believe it or not, you can actually train your child to comply through simple repetition. Just as how fast you learn an exercise routine depends a lot on how often you perform the workout, how well your child acquires the compliance habit depends on how often he or she has a chance to practice. The second technique to use this week is to establish a schedule of "cooperation workouts."

1. Find at least two or three times a day when your child is not very busy and is not intensely occupied with fun activities that the child will hate interrupting. For a young child with a predictable routine, these can be roughly the same times every day; with an older child, you'll have to watch for opportunities.

2. Now begin giving a series of five or six commands over the next three to five minutes. *Keep the commands extremely simple and easy to follow:* "Please hand me that book"; "Can you reach that pencil on the table for me?"; "Close the curtain on that window, please"; "Turn on that lamp"; and so forth. Each command should require only very brief, minimal effort from your child.

3. As your child complies with each request, praise him or her as you would for obeying ordinary requests given in the course of your day.

- *Very young children can be rewarded with a small taste of a favorite food or drink.*
- *For older children, verbal appreciation should be enough.*

Give Compelling Commands

In my years of work with defiant children, I have found that simply altering the way you give commands and make requests can greatly improve your child's response. This week, while you're sticking around to follow through on commands so you can praise your child for cooperating, also work on shaping your commands for the best effect. Here are six steps and two tools to help you do this:

Six Steps

1. *Make Sure You Mean It.* A lot of parents greet this advice with indignation or incredulity: "Do you really think I'd put myself in the position of making *unnecessary* demands of a kid who doesn't obey anyway?" I know you're not aware of making superfluous requests of your child—and that's the point. While some parents of defiant children get so discouraged that they simply abdicate—they stop paying attention and making requests at all—others get into the habit of making too many demands. The reasons are not entirely clear. Maybe it's an unconscious form of experimentation—"Let's throw everything we've got at this problem and see what sticks"—to identify *which* commands are a problem. Or it could be just a desperate attempt to feel better about your own competence by getting your child to obey *some* command.

In any case, unless you're willing to follow through as instructed in this chapter, giving extra commands just gives your child and you more opportunities to "fail." Therefore, the first thing you need to do when giving normal, everyday commands this week is to stop yourself and think about the relative importance of the command before you issue it. Is this a high priority? Is it something your child has to do right now? And most important, are you willing to stick around and follow through? *If the answer to any of these questions is no, don't say anything.* Postpone the job or forget about it altogether. *If the answer is yes, be prepared to back up whatever you ask with both positive and negative consequences.* As time goes on and your child begins to understand that you mean every command you give, compliance will grow.

2. *Tell, Don't Ask.* Lee, in the "before" scenario at the beginning of this chapter, immediately shot herself in the foot when she phrased her command to Norm in the form of a question, as if she were requesting a favor. That kind of wording immediately tells the child he or she has the option of refusing to comply. You don't have to be rude (you can still say "please" as Lee did in the "after" scenario), and once your child

has developed a solid habit of complying, you can return to extra niceties. For now, though, make your request a simple statement.

3. *Keep It Simple.* Almost all children, especially younger ones, will get confused by a complicated command or several at once. The usual response to this confusion is to comply with none of what you've asked. Stick to one command at a time even if you need your child to complete several tasks. Wait until you've praised the child for successfully completing the first one before imposing the next. If what you're asking is complex, do your best to break it down into several simpler steps to be accomplished and praised separately (see the tools that follow).

4. *Make Sure You Are Heard.* Without eye contact, you can't really be sure your child has listened. Many of us fall prey to the temptation to shout an order from another room or to continue with what we're doing without looking up while issuing a command. If necessary, gently turn your child's face toward you to be sure he or she has paid attention.

5. *Get Rid of the Competition.* Another way to make sure the child is hearing you is to eliminate all other distractions—TV, stereo, video games, or anything else that's likely to compete strongly for the child's attention. You can tell your child to turn off these interferences, but many parents prefer to do it themselves so they don't have to issue a command before they even get to the point.

6. *Make Sure You Are Understood.* If you don't think the child has both heard and understood what you want—the child stares at you unblinkingly, has a vague look on his or her face, does not reply, or makes no eye contact with you, ask the child to repeat the command. This seems especially helpful in enhancing compliance from children with a short attention span, such as those with ADHD.

Two Helpful Tools

1. *Use a Timer.* Any reminder you can give the child that "time is of the essence" will help the child get going, so many parents find it

extremely helpful to tell the child how much time is being allowed for completion of the task and then set a timer for that period. If you choose to do this, of course, follow-up is necessary. What will the child earn for completing the task within the allotted time? What penalties will be imposed for not doing so? As Lee showed in the "after" scenario, sometimes the incentive that you offer can keep the child moving toward the next task you have in mind.

2. *Make Up Chore Cards.* For children who are old enough to read and to be assigned regular chores or other tasks, making up chore cards helps the child stay on track and also prevents any debates about what you meant when you asked your daughter, for example, to "clean up the kitchen after dinner." Using three-by-five-inch file cards, simply write down the steps necessary to do the job you want done, in order. The child can carry the card around as a reminder while doing the task. Some parents find it helpful to add the time limit for the whole job (or even for the individual steps in it) and to use the timer along with the chore cards.

Reducing Interruptions

"All day I could have used some help with chores and errands, and Nicky was nowhere to be found. When I had time to go over his homework with him, he had magically disappeared. Why is it that the only time he seems to be all over me is when I'm trying to make a phone call, pay some bills, or read a book?"

Complaints about the inability to get things done without interruption are a common lament among parents with defiant children. Being unable to talk on the phone, do paperwork, converse at the dinner table, read, or watch TV without constant interruption geometrically increases the frustration of having your commands refused, your admonitions ignored, and your wishes resisted.

On the surface, behavior like Nicky's does seem paradoxical. It's not so hard to understand, though, when you view it as another facet of the attention issue. In that light, it's not impossible to change, either.

Your child persists in interrupting your conversations and disrupting your work because he gets attention for doing so—and no attention for leav-

---

SAMPLE CHORE CARD

The following is a card created for 10-year-old Maria.

Job: Clean up after dinner
Time: 20 minutes

1. Clear the table. 5 minutes
2. Scrape the plates. 5 minutes
3. Put away the leftovers. 5 minutes
4. Load the dishwasher. 5 minutes

Reward for finishing: ½ hour TV time
Reward for finishing in 20 minutes: 1 hour TV time

---

ing you alone. Maybe you scold or yell at your child when he keeps bugging you while you're trying to cook dinner. Perhaps you even cut short your phone calls when little Danielle refuses to stop screaming in your other ear while you're talking to a friend. Or maybe you and your spouse finally get exasperated when your young son won't let you catch up on the events of each other's day at the dinner table: "All *right,* Bobby, why don't you tell us about *your* day if you really can't wait."

The solution should be obvious: Make it more appealing to the child to leave you alone. Pay attention when the child is not interrupting and do your best to ignore the child's attempt to butt in. The technique involves practice in giving the child something to do while you're occupied and periodically interrupting *yourself* to praise the child for not interrupting you. Over the next week, follow these steps, gradually increasing the time between offerings of praise so that you gain gradually longer times to do what you need to do.

1. Whenever you know you're about to make a phone call of some length, start on some job that requires your undivided concentration, or just have some peaceful downtime, come up with an enjoyable activity and tell your child to do that while you're busy and not to interrupt you.

2. Now start on your activity, but stop what you're doing after about 30 seconds and praise your child for succeeding in not interrupting you.

3. Return to your activity, this time stopping after about a minute to praise your child for not interrupting you.

4. Continue this pattern, increasing the intervals between offerings of praise, until you're finished.

- *Pick two or three particularly troublesome activities to practice this technique with over the week. Many parents find phone calls a real problem. If you target phone calls, consider having a friend or your spouse call you at home a couple of times a day so you can practice the exercise without offending the person on the other end of the call.*

- *The activity you use to occupy your child should not be elaborate or unusual but should definitely be something the child enjoys, whether it's coloring, watching TV, or playing a video game. It should never be a chore.*

- *If you can tell that your child is about to stop whatever she's doing to come over and interrupt you, immediately stop what you're doing and go over to the child to praise her for not interrupting.*

- *You can increase the intervals between praises not only within one session but also from session to session during the week.*

- *The praise you offer the child at the end of this period should be greater than the periodic praises you've been giving throughout the task. Consider a small reward on top of verbal praise.*

- *This practice should continue until your child, depending on maturity, can play independently for about 10 minutes. Remember, however, that your initial goal is not to complete the task you need to do but to pay attention and praise your child for not interrupting.*

Knowing What Your Child Is Up To

Research suggests that the behavior and social conduct of defiant children tends to disintegrate across the board when parents fail to monitor the child. That is, it's not just when you want compliance or peace and quiet from your child that your child needs attention from you. It's true that you probably hear more protests and have more conflict with your child than anyone else because you have to make the most demands of the child, but that doesn't mean the rest of the child's life

MAKING A PHONE CALL: THE RIGHT WAY
AND THE WRONG WAY

The Wrong Kind of Attention

"Danny, I'm going to call Daddy at the office. If you interrupt me, you're going to start your naptime a whole hour early." ... [Mom dials phone.]

"Hi, honey, it's me. I just wanted to let you know I might not be here when you—hang on a minute, honey...."

"Danny, turn down that TV this minute. I can't hear a word Daddy's saying!"

"Sorry, honey—I just don't know what I'm going to do with that boy. So, about this evening—"

"Danny! Put that down this instant! You know you're not allowed to use Mommy's scissors."

"I better make this fast—"

"What? No, you can't have a snack. You just had breakfast."

"OK, so—"

"DANNY! Close that refrigerator! I said no snack right now!!"

"What I'm trying to tell you—oh, hold on...."

"OK, Mister, you're going to be quiet while I talk to Daddy if I

The Right Kind of Attention

"Danny, I'm going to call Daddy at the office. I want you to color this picture of the doggy while I'm on the phone. Don't interrupt me."

"Hi, honey, it's me. I just wanted to let you know I might not be here when you get home. [Mom sees Danny start to get up from table.] Hang on a minute, honey...."

"Danny, I'm so proud of you for letting me talk to Daddy. Keep it up!" [Danny plunks back down into chair.]

"Sorry, honey. Anyway, I have to take Danny to the dentist, and we might be late. Hold on one more time, OK?"

"Danny, you're doing such a good job. Thanks for being so helpful!" [Leans over and kisses the top of Danny's head.]

"So, if we're not back by the time you get here, can you take the casserole out of the refrigerator and put it in the oven? It has to go in for an hour at 350, so just set the timer, and I'll check when I get home.... One more time ..."

"Wow, Danny, you're terrific. Keep coloring, please."

(cont.)

The Wrong Kind of Attention	The Right Kind of Attention
have to sit on you!" [Mom grabs Danny's hand and holds him next to her while she picks up the phone again.] "Anyway, I might not be home . . . what? Oh, Grace, it's you. What? He had to go? OK, [sighs] I'll call him back later." *"Danny Johnson, you march right up to your room and stay there until I come up and decide what to do with you!"*	"I'm a little worried about Danny's molars, so I plan to talk to Dr. Greene about them. We may have to go back for another check on them soon, but next time I'll try to make it earlier in the morning. As you know, late afternoon isn't Danny's best time of day. Oh, well. I'll see if I can get him to take a little longer nap first. Boy, he's really hanging in there right now. Maybe you should mention it when you get home. Well, I'll let you get back to work. See you later!" *"Danny, you are such a great help to me when you let me finish my phone calls. Daddy and I are so proud of you. How would you like to play a quick game of Chutes and Ladders before lunch?"*

is Camelot. Unless friends and neighbors, brothers and sisters, classmates, and other adults in authoritative positions are willing and able to defer to your child's every wish, trouble can brew anywhere. So your job doesn't end with your face-to-face encounters with your child. *You need to interrupt your own activities periodically during the day to check on your child when he or she is not within your sight.* Running up to a sibling's room and complimenting your defiant child for playing so cooperatively can increase the amount of time your child is able to hold it together with others. Ditto for playing out in the neighborhood. Although this may seem like a burden at first, it doesn't really take much time. The tough part is remembering to do it regularly. Here again, a timer or a watch with an alarm that can be set to regular intervals is a great help.

• *Even if you use a timer, try not to make your monitoring too predictable. A child can put on an innocent mask in a second if he knows he'll be called on to do so at certain intervals.*

• *If you find the child misbehaving when you check up on her, deliver your usual discipline swiftly.*

• *Please don't neglect this part of Step 2. Our research shows that parental monitoring of a child's activities is one of the most critical determinants of which children drift into deviant and antisocial behavior.*

Trouble Spots and Stumbling Blocks

"Our pediatrician has always instructed us not to use food as a reward, because treating food as more than sustenance can be the beginning of eating disorders. Why do you recommend snacks and treats as rewards for compliance?"

There is no evidence from research that using occasional snack food rewards encourages obesity or eating disorders. If you're concerned about it, just be sure to use small tastes of the treat or snack, not bagfuls. Also, try using more nutritious snacks as rewards, though clearly they must still be desirable to the child.

"I'd like nothing more than to praise my child for not interrupting my phone calls, but I have yet to see 15 seconds pass without his babbling at me. How can I get this exercise started if he never leaves me alone long enough to earn any praise?"

Try starting with a different situation in which you don't want to be interrupted, such as preparing dinner, trying to talk to your spouse, or just trying to read a magazine.

"Nothing I started this week seemed to work. I did my best to praise James for behaving well—though about the only place where I could do this regularly was in not interrupting me—and I tried holding compliance practice sessions, but usually he found a reason to get away from me. Why aren't these techniques making him do what I ask?"

Praise just takes a long time to sink in with some kids. Please be patient and keep it up over the next few weeks. First, be sure what you're offering really is praise and not some offhanded or backhanded statement. Second, for kids with severe problems with defiance, praise simply may not be enough; but keep it up anyway, because it will support all your future efforts (and make you feel better). Rest assured that in the next step you'll be introduced to a technique that is even more potent than praise in encouraging compliance.

Also, please try to remain focused this week on changing your own behavior, not your child's. That is your primary goal; changes in your child's behavior will follow.

"My daughter is a smart, skeptical nine-year-old who takes nothing at face value. When I suddenly started praising her for every little cooperative effort, and especially for not interrupting me, she just scowled at me and went on as usual. Now she's starting to ask what I'm up to. How can I be truthful about what I'm doing without making her feel manipulated? She'd resist that more than anything else."

Many parents find it difficult to put these techniques into effect without sounding unnatural, and that unease shows in how they behave toward their children at first. Very few parents have trouble understanding the importance of praise or the workings of the techniques in Step 2, but many find they're not as easy as they sounded once they start putting them into practice. All I can say is that it will get easier with time. When your typical dialogue with your child is acerbic, the transition to complimenting the child for doing what you want is tough. This is a time when you have to be particularly vigilant to avoid making your praise sound sarcastic or turning it into backhanded compliments.

Remember why you're doing any of this—because you love and want to help your child—and try any honest heartfelt response. You might simply say, "I'm trying to change the way I act so it's easier for you and me to get along." One little boy asked his mother if she'd gone crazy when she started complimenting him for not interrupting her. Her answer satisfied him completely: "No, it's just that I don't think I let you know often enough when you're doing a great job."

"Jeanette just ignored me, as she always does, when I tried the compliance practice sessions with her. I felt pretty stupid continuing to make trivial

requests of her when she didn't even bother to look up at me. Am I doing something wrong?"

No. In fact, if you're ignoring her ignoring you, you're doing everything right. If this keeps up for the whole three to five minutes you've allotted, just try again later, perhaps when your daughter already seems to be more receptive, such as when she's already talking amiably with you. Having their attention at the start sometimes makes kids comply with simple requests before they have a chance to think about it.

If all else fails, try this brilliant idea from one mother: Tina reported that her son never did anything the first time she asked, and so she wasn't having much luck with the compliance practice exercise. That all turned around when she tried this set of requests during one session: "Get yourself a Coke," "Get yourself some cookies," "Serve yourself some ice cream." Boy, was her son receptive the next time around!

"My daughter interrupts virtually everything I do. She may not do much of what I ask, but she never goes away. She stands around and chatters or whines at me constantly. If I don't respond, she starts tugging at my clothes and even hitting me. I don't even know where to begin with the exercise for not interrupting."

In a case like that, it's really crucial to set your priorities—and start slowly. Don't, for instance, start by tackling the hour you have to spend once a week on household paperwork. Instead, pick a typically brief activity. One mother decided that the activity she most wanted to work on not having interrupted was having some privacy in the bathroom!

"I think I've done a pretty good job of putting your instructions into effect on giving better commands, but I'm still not getting much response. I tell my son not to talk with his mouth full, and he just grins at me and keeps on going. I tell him to stop stomping across the floor, and he gets louder. I tell him to stop teasing his sister, and he just does it more sneakily. What can I do?"

Take another look at the list of commands you just mentioned—they're all negatives. Sometimes the best way to refigure your commands is to turn them into positives. One father I advised was very surprised to see the difference it made when he told his son what he wanted him to do rather than what he wanted him not to do. He used to say, for example, "Don't leave your sneakers in the middle of the living room floor," and later he would find the sneakers in the middle of the dining room floor. When he said instead, "Put your sneakers in the closet," that's where they ended up.

When you talk to your son, instead of "Don't talk with your mouth full," try "Please finish that bite, then talk." Instead of "Don't stomp across the floor," say "Take your shoes off while you're in the house so your feet don't make so much noise." Instead of "Stop bugging your sister," try either "Go do something by yourself for the next 15 minutes" or "Cindy will probably be happy to play with you if you bring out the pick-up-sticks game."

"We've had some success with modifying the way we ask our daughter to do things, but certain commands still fall on deaf ears, and I can't figure out why. Help!"

Review those things she absolutely refuses to do. First, be sure your daughter is actually capable of doing what you've asked. Some parents assign tasks that are far above their child's developmental level. Second, are you sure she understands exactly what you want? Some parents just don't get specific enough, and their children are therefore unable, not unwilling, to comply. When one couple got frustrated by their son's refusal to "Get off the computer by supper time" as they consistently asked, they came upon a solution when they finally, through observation, realized that he got so engrossed in the computer that he lost track of time and didn't realize when it was supper time. The problem disappeared when they bought a big clock with a timer on it that they set up on top of the computer.

"I haven't been able to bring myself to compliment my daughter for not interrupting while I'm on the phone, because in my experience it's better with her to 'let sleeping dogs lie.' Whenever I tried in the past to reward her

*for playing on her own, she immediately acted up. Why should I believe it
will work this time?"*

How did you behave when your child acted up in those circumstances? You probably stayed in the room with her and gave her a lecture or paid some other attention that negatively reinforced her misbehavior. She simply learned that she could keep your attention longer
by requiring a scolding. In this exercise, you simply ignore the misbehavior—leave the room entirely—to discourage the acting up.

Also, be aware that if you don't start rewarding your child's independent play, it will never increase beyond the frequency that you see
now. In fact, it will probably diminish over time because the child will
get discouraged when you don't notice and appreciate it. Please try
this; it works.

*"It doesn't make sense to me to interrupt myself so that my child won't
interrupt me. How will I ever get anything done?"*

It's true that at first you'll have to keep disrupting your own activities to instill the lessons of this exercise. If this is a serious problem
for you, then try limiting the exercise to less important activities—but
still those you don't want interrupted—such as social phone calls or
tasks that are not urgent to complete right away. Regardless of which
activities you target, it shouldn't take more than a few days before
your uninterrupted periods increase substantially if you've been following the instructions and gradually increasing periods between offerings of praise to your child.

*"Can't I put off checking on my child while he's not in the room for another
week? I already feel like I'm losing a tremendous amount of time doing the
other parts of Step 2. This one doesn't seem as important."*

Ignorance is bliss, I guess. Many parents—of both defiant and
nondefiant children—don't have a clue about what their children are
up to when they're not in plain view. All children sometimes show a
different face when they're not being supervised, and of course we
parents all hope that the lessons we impart stay with them even when
we're not there to enforce them. With defiant children, though, it

would be unrealistic to expect too much in this area. As I mentioned in describing the exercise, there are just too many temptations, too many situations that will push the child's buttons. You'll really be helping your child improve other relationships if you occasionally check on how things are going. Besides, research has shown that inadequate monitoring is a major contributor to antisocial behaviors like stealing, lying, vandalism, and other clandestine activities. You can save yourself a lot of heartache in the future if you just get in the habit of keeping an eye on your child now.

CHAPTER 7

Step 3: When Praise Is Not Enough, Offer Rewards

Before . . .

"Let's see if you can get that math done in 20 minutes, Lenny. I'll set the timer."

Lenny plunked down into his chair at the desk and pulled his math worksheet toward him with a heavy sigh. His mother watched from a chair in the corner of his room until she saw him pick up his pencil, then she looked back down at her book.

About two minutes later, Kathy looked up again and said quietly, "I'm proud of you for concentrating so hard, Len."

Her son smiled but kept at his homework.

A couple of minutes later, Kathy heard Lenny shifting in his seat, scuffing his feet on the floor, and rustling his papers around on his desk. Quickly she looked up and said, "Great job, Len. Keep it up."

The noises continued, but Lenny stayed with his work.

Another few minutes passed, and now Lenny was clearing his throat and tapping his pencil on the desk. Kathy prompted, "You must be making great progress on that math. Don't give up now—you're terrific!"

The next time Kathy looked up from her reading it was because the noises from Len's desk had stopped abruptly. Now he was gazing out the window with a dreamy look on his face. Kathy walked over to the desk and said, "I see you're halfway there, Len. Good job!"

Her son went back to his work, and the same pattern continued until the timer rang.

Kathy stood up to check Lenny's work. He had completed only one more problem since he started to stare out the window. "That's OK, honey, you really did a good job. Let's see if we can finish this up."

Reluctantly, Kathy laid her book down on her son's bed and pulled her chair up to his desk. "Now, let's see. . . ."

Twenty minutes later, with his mother right by his side, Lenny had finished his math homework. Downstairs in the living room, her husband asked her how it had gone.

"Same as always, I guess," she answered. "He gets it done, and we don't get into too many major battles over it anymore, but I'm not sure which one of us should be getting the report card this quarter. He can't seem to get his work done without me hovering over him every minute. I'm beginning to feel like I have no life at all—I'm just Lenny's shadow."

After . . .

"Let's see if you can get that math done in 20 minutes, Lenny. I'll set the timer, and if you finish it before the bell rings, you'll get 10 points. Remember that Bulls jersey you're working for!"

Before she left the room, Kathy tapped the Bulls insignia on the wall chart over her son's desk. It showed the number of points Lenny could earn for completing various tasks and the number of points he needed to get various rewards and privileges.

A minute later, Kathy quietly poked her head back through the door to make sure her son was working on his math. Lenny seemed to be concentrating hard. His mother watched him look back up at the chart and timer every time he finished a problem, just like she'd taught him.

"Good job, Len!" she said, giving him a thumbs-up sign and a big smile before slipping out again.

Ten minutes later—Kathy had her own timer by her side in the living room—she looked in on her son again. His knee was jiggling madly under his desk, and she heard him say to himself, "Come on, only three more problems to go. Let's go!" Quietly his mother tapped the Bulls logo on the chart and said, "Don't worry, Len. I know you're going to do it. Terrific work!"

Her son smiled up at her before she left.

Kathy had set her timer for a total of 18 minutes so she'd be sure to be in Len's room when his 20 minutes were up. She walked into his room just in time to see him throw his pencil up in the air and yell, "Two points!"

"No, that's 10 points, Len, and, boy, am I proud of you!" Kathy pulled a pen from her pocket and with a flourish added a 10 to the "deposit" column in a notebook labeled "Lenny's Bank Book."

"That's 30 points today just for getting all your homework done on time, honey. So what's it gonna be—TV? A bike ride?"

"I'm going to use 20 on TV and put 10 toward the Bulls shirt," Len announced.

"Great," said his mother, then she gave him a high five and left.

If you feel like Kathy in the "before" scenario, you would probably agree that Step 2 was time well spent. Your child still may not behave well unsupervised, but the changes you've made in your *own* behavior should have made noticeable inroads into the problems between you. Perhaps now your son *does* get his homework done, if only with you as stalwart cheerleader and tutor. Maybe your daughter *doesn't* stomp out of the room when you make the simplest request of her, because now you make a supreme effort to keep the "I know you're going to fight me on this" tone out of your voice. If so, you should take satisfaction from knowing you've done what you set out to do in Step 2: Reframe your part of the dialogue when you need cooperation from your child.

As a result, your relationship should be friendlier, not just during "special time" but when you're going about your daily business together, too. The combination of earning your favor and getting lots of practice in doing what you ask may make arguing for the sake of arguing less appealing to your child. And now that you're issuing commands only when you really mean them, the two of you should have even fewer opportunities for confrontation.

Of course you don't want to settle for that. No parent wants to feel the way Kathy feels—like a sentinel who never goes off duty. Fortunately, you have another incentive to offer your child for cooperating without constant supervision. In Step 3, you'll learn how to give your child rewards for behaving appropriately—not just praise and attention but tangible treats and privileges that your child holds dear.

You may already have an inkling of how powerful a motivator rewards can be because many of you have already been handing out little snacks or toys along with the kudos to reinforce notable achievements in your child's behavior. Systematize the reward process, and it becomes a formidable tool indeed. *More than half of the families I've ushered through this program have seen their child's behavior problems disappear almost entirely after Step 3.*

Why do some kids, like Lenny, need this extra push? As you know, few kids are defiant solely because they've learned to act that way. Many have inborn trouble paying attention and controlling their impulses. Therefore, changing your behavior, as you learned to do in Step 2, may make it easier for them to fight their nature at the moment, but it won't erase the traits that make it hard for them to look ahead and defer gratification independently. To persuade them to form the habit of sacrificing what they'd prefer to do right now in favor of what you want them to do, you have to give them something to look forward to. In other words, there had better be a carrot on the end of that stick.

You don't have to delve too far into your own experience to understand how effective rewards are. How often have you given up the evening at home that you want right now for the prospect of a bonus at the end of the year? Who among us has not found the will to push away a slice of cheesecake tonight for better-fitting clothes tomorrow? Noncompliant children are no different. They just need their rewards to be more frequent, more immediate, and more concrete. That's what Step 3 will give them: a way to earn points toward "prizes" numerous times a day so that they can see themselves getting ever closer to something they want very much.

Not surprisingly, this is a tool that everyone can use, and *I strongly recommend that you adopt it with any defiant child of age four or over, even if your child has already made great strides with Step 2.* This reward system will speed up the progress your child is making, can nudge your child's behavior all the way into the normal range, and can make those improvements permanent, even after you stop using the system.

If your child is three or younger, please stick to immediate, tangible rewards for compliance, such as giving the child a small snack, a sticker, or a little toy or playing a brief game together. Little children may not be able to grasp the concept that chips or points stand for rewards and privileges. Even if they do, their number skills are bound to make this exercise difficult.

What you'll be doing this week is setting up a token system whereby your child earns chips or points for completing certain tasks when asked and can then redeem these tokens for rewards or privileges the child values. Why can't you just simplify matters and slip the child a little something on the spot, as you sometimes do now? When you hand out the number of rewards that it takes to encourage positive behavior, little snacks and tiny treats quickly lose their appeal—and, therefore, their power to motivate. You need a variety of rewards, some of them bigger than others, and most of these cannot practically be awarded on the spot. You can't reward the completion of math homework with 15 minutes of TV when your child still has science and reading assignments ahead of him. Nor would you want to reward your child for 10 minutes of not interrupting your writing by interrupting yourself to play a 30-minute game with her. The answer is to keep the child motivated by *immediately* giving points for compliance—a reward that's tangible enough to be motivating and can be redeemed later for a specific privilege.

Sounds like a game, doesn't it? It should. The whole project should be undertaken with a positive tone and introduced as something enjoyable as well as constructive. Make it fun and get creative with props, and your child will enter into the program with the same enthusiasm.

For 4- to 7-year-olds, you'll award poker chips (or some other small token) for compliance; for 8- to 12-year-olds, you can use a written point system instead. Either way, the system is easy to implement throughout the day. Follow these steps:

The Home Poker Chip Program: Ages Four to Seven

1. Get a standard set of plastic poker chips—many households already have one. If your child is only four or five years old, the white, red, and blue chips will all count as one chip or point. If your child is six or seven, you can use the chips the way you would in poker: white = 1, blue = 5, and red = 10. In that case, tape one chip of each color to a card and label the value of each color; you'll give this to your child as a reminder.

2. Find a quiet time to explain the system to your child. To keep the tone positive, tell your child that you don't think the child has been rewarded enough for all the good things he or she does at home. To change that, you're going to start awarding chips for behaving well so the child can earn rewards and privileges that he or she likes. Make it clear right away that you'll be setting up a firm plan so both of you will always know what to expect from each other. Tell your son or daughter that he or she will be allowed to help make up the list of rewards that can be earned.

3. Show your child the poker chips and explain that these will be the "money" earned for doing certain jobs and that he or she will earn different numbers of chips for different jobs: The harder and longer the job, the more chips earned. State up front that the child will earn chips only for doing the job upon your first request and only when the job is finished. "If I have to ask you twice to make your bed," you might say, "you'll still have to make your bed, but you won't get any chips for it." Or, "I asked you to make your bed, and it's great that you went in there to do it right away, but you didn't finish, so you don't get any chips this time."

4. Together, decide on a "bank" that can be used to hold the chips: a coffee can with a dull rim, a shoebox, a plastic jar, or another container. Let the child help designate the bank. Then the two of you can have some fun decorating it.

5. Now make up a list of privileges: Ask your child what he or she would like to earn for behaving well. Most kids will start with the biggies, like a favorite outing or something they know they don't get very often because it's expensive or inconvenient. Go ahead and list these, but make sure you add everyday privileges as well. Aim for 10 to 15 privileges, one-third of them short term, one-third middle term, and one-third long term. For example:

- Five short-term privileges: watching TV, playing a video game, using roller blades, riding a bike, having a friend over after school
- Five middle-term privileges: staying up past bedtime, watching a special one-time TV program, spending the night at a

friend's home, baking cookies with Mom or Dad, choosing the family's dinner menu
- Five long-term privileges: going to a restaurant for dinner, renting a video, having a party with friends, going to an amusement park, buying a sports-team jersey

6. Now make a list of tasks to be done to earn chips. These can be everyday personal tasks such as brushing teeth and getting dressed, chores such as setting the table and taking out the garbage, responsibilities such as completing homework and feeding the dog, and social conduct such as not hitting a younger sibling or sharing toys with a visiting friend. A few important guidelines:

- The child should participate in making this list, but you should have the final say in what is included.
- Look back at the questionnaires in Chapter 1 and the ADHD questionnaire in Chapter 2. If the problem areas that you identified on those forms have changed at all, fill them out again. Use the current forms to remind yourself of the areas in which your child's behavior is the greatest problem. If washing and bathing are big issues, list these personal tasks so that you can encourage your child to carry them out. If arguing with adults is a major problem, list not arguing with adults as a goal to be rewarded.
- If you are going to list things you want your child *not* to do, be prepared to establish a time period during which the child has to forgo that behavior to earn points—for example, not arguing with an adult between breakfast and lunch.
- *Be sure to tell your child that you will sometimes—but not always— give bonus chips when he or she does a job promptly or with a particularly pleasant attitude.*

7. Now assign the number of chips that can be earned for each of these jobs. For younger kids—ages four and five—stick to one to three chips for each task, perhaps five for a really big job such as picking up all their toys in the family room or playroom. Kids aged six and seven can earn 1 to 10 points for each task, in recognition of the higher level of difficulty of responsibility.

8. Now determine how many chips the child will have to pay you for each privilege listed. This is a job for you alone. Start by roughly adding up how many chips you think the child will earn in a typical day. I usually advise parents to make sure that about two-thirds of the chips earned that day can be spent on privileges that will be used that day. That way the child can save up the other third for longer term privileges. Don't worry too much about precision at this point. Just be sure to charge more chips for larger rewards than for the daily privileges and try to be fair.

Here is a sample chart for a five- or six-year-old child who might earn 30 chips per day on a weekday:

Privilege	Cost
TV (½ hour)	3 (limit: 2 hours/schoolday)
Video/computer games (½ hour)	3 (limit: 1 hour/schoolday)
Play outdoors	1
Ride bike	1
Choose special dessert from pantry	1
Stay up past bedtime with parents' permission	3 (per ½ hour)
Have a friend over to play	5
Go to a friend's house to play	5
Rent a video game or movie	20
Go out for fast food (child chooses)	30
Spend the night at a friend's	30
Go to the movies	50
Buy a special toy/item	Varies (1 chip = 20 cents)
Allowance: $2 per week	10

Note that the child needs 20 chips to get typical daily privileges. To be fair, when in doubt, keep it cheap. That is, if you aren't sure about a price, err on the low side so the child will see it as reasonable. This is easier than it may sound before you've tried it. Once you see about how much your child can earn in a typical day, you get a feel for what might be fair. For instance, if a child is earning 30 chips a day, and we want to be sure he spends 20 of them on daily privileges, should a half-hour of TV cost 20 chips? Of course not. But it should not cost only 1 chip either, because that would let the child have 10 hours of TV! Parents tend to gravitate toward something like three chips per half-hour of TV or Nintendo time. Also, we want kids to do some things for their own good, like play outside when it is a nice day, so we might charge them only one or two chips for that privilege.

Think of the first week as a shakedown cruise, meaning you will discover whether your assignment of chips is reasonable and then can change it as the program plays out. Some adjustments will be made during the first week or so, but most families I have counseled have not found setting up a fair reward–privilege scale too difficult. Remember too that your child can have a say in the adjustments that are made so his or her opinions have some influence on the program.

9. Remind the child of how chips can be earned: for doing a job the first time you ask, as a bonus for a great attitude, and for other good behavior that you and the child have not listed, such as for not bothering you while you work or not interrupting you while on the phone.

IS IT A RIGHT OR A PRIVILEGE?

Talking about rewards and privileges naturally appeals to children who are accustomed to discussions that center on punishment and penalties. Despite this enthusiasm, the process has its pitfalls. Here are a few caveats to keep in mind:

Make sure you include a range of privileges. Kids have no trouble conjuring up their wildest dreams to include on the list. You may need to fill in the other end of the list, balancing the trips to amusement parks and expensive toy purchases with the little privileges like watching TV, choosing a short game to play with Mom or Dad (or both), or having a friend over after school. There are two reasons for this: (1) You want the child to have to earn privileges every day so the child will be more motivated to behave, and (2) you want the child to have constant reminders of successes achieved.

Distinguish carefully between rights and privileges to make the system fair. The child should never be charged for necessities like food,

(cont.)

---

shelter, clothing, or a hug—these are the child's rights in the most fundamental sense. Beyond that, however, where the line is drawn between a right and a privilege varies from family to family and child to child. In one of our parent training groups an interesting difference arose regarding Little League. One couple believed that participating in Little League was their son's right. That is, they would never charge for it because they would never take it away from him—it was very important to them to see him engage in a positive social activity. Another couple in the group felt that Little League was a privilege because it demanded much time and expense on their part; these parents decided it was correct to charge the boy poker chips for each practice.

Be creative. If your list contains too little variety, your child will quickly lose interest in trying to earn the privileges. Don't limit your list to what your child already enjoys; use your imagination to come up with new possibilities. Other parents have found these ideas intriguing to kids: a chance to try the latest breakfast cereals, choosing a baseball card from a big stack, pulling a surprise out of a grab bag, and painting fingernails.

Anticipate how often a child might choose a listed reward and impose time limits if necessary. In one family, selecting what was served for supper was included in the list of privileges to be earned, but after a week of macaroni and cheese, pizza, and hot dogs, the parents decided to limit this option to once a week!

Once you're sure the child understands the program, say you'll start the plan the next day. *When you do so, the most important thing to keep in mind this first week is to be especially generous in giving away chips. The program will fail instantly if the child cannot easily earn chips and thus privileges. No chips = no rewards = no incentive to behave well!*

The Home Point System: Ages 8 through 12

Use this token program for children aged 8 through 12. It's a little more sophisticated and involves bigger responsibilities and commensurately larger numbers of points earned and probably a broader range of rewards, too. Because you use a simple notebook rather than a poker chip bank, this version is particularly mobile, which most parents find helpful with the more peripatetic third- through seventh-graders (using the program away from home will be discussed in Chapter 10). Set up the program this way:

1. Buy a standard 8½-by-11-inch notebook and label the front to identify it as your child's home point record. Again, you and the child—or the child alone—can decorate it to give it added importance. Set up five columns as in a standard checkbook: date, item, deposit, withdrawal, balance. Explain to your child that whenever he or she has earned a reward for compliance, you'll enter the date, a short description of the job or behavior in the "item" column, the number of points earned in the "deposit" column, and then the new balance in that column. Whenever the child spends points to get a reward or privilege, you'll enter the amount used up in the "withdrawal" column and subtract that amount to get a new balance in the last column. *Tell your child that only you will be making entries in the book; the child may not do so.*

2. With your child, make up a list of rewards and privileges in the same way as described for the poker chip program. Obviously, this list will reflect the child's greater age.

3. Now make up a list of jobs as described for the chip program. Because an older child will probably be more able to help with household chores than a younger child, some of the tasks you include will likely be more complicated and take a longer time.

4. Now assign numbers of points earned for each job on behavior. Again, because the jobs are likely harder than for younger kids, assign larger numbers of points. I typically recommend 5 to 25 points for routine daily jobs and up to 200 points for very big ones. One guideline you can start with is 15 points for every 15 minutes of work, whether it's a chore around the house or homework. For behavior you're trying to discourage, it's typical to give fewer points per time period, such as 5 points for 15 minutes of avoiding misbehavior. That depends, however, on how hard it is for your child to resist the designated misbehavior. The more difficult you perceive that impulse control to be for your child, the more points you should award for success.

5. As explained in the chip program, figure about how many points your child is likely to earn in a day to determine how much each privilege should cost. Again, make sure the child will be able to save up about one-third of the points earned in a day toward larger future rewards.

Put the plan into effect just as you would for the chip program.

Jmportant Dos and Don'ts for the Token Systems

- *Don't* introduce the program by telling the child that because he or she always misbehaves, you're taking away all of his or her privileges and he or she will have to earn them back again.
- *Don't* fine the child by deducting chips or points for misbehavior. This program is to be used at this stage only to give the child incentive for good behavior.
- *Don't* be stingy with chips during this first week; reward even the tiniest good behavior.
- *Do* make sure both parents use the program.
- *Don't* give any chips or points if you have to repeat a command.
- *Don't* give the child chips or points until he or she has finished the job.
- *Don't* wait to reward the child—give him or her the chips or points immediately following completion of the task.
- *Do* reinforce the reward with praise—smile when you give out chips or points!
- *Do* be specific about what the child did to earn the chips or points, even though the task is recorded on your list—say what you liked about what the child just did.

Making Jt Work: Jnnovative Tips from Parents

Try these tried-and-true ideas to enhance either the poker chip or the point system.

- Prereaders will be motivated to earn chips if you make up separate charts for the rewards and the jobs that use pictures to represent these items and tasks. Try cutting pictures out of magazines.
- All kids benefit from reminders. Consider dividing up the tasks you're targeting and posting little reminder charts in places where those tasks are usually done. Examples:

In the bathroom:	Over the desk:
Brush teeth: 3 points	Finish math sheet in 20 minutes: 10 points
Put toothpaste away: 2 points	Finish book report in 1 hour: 60 points
Brush hair: 3 points	Reading assignments: Finish 1 page in 5 minutes: 5 points
Wash face: 3 points	
Hang up towels: 2 points	Studying for tests: For every 15 minutes: 15 points

- For younger kids, substitute chips for points and use only pictures (a picture of a toothbrush means brushing teeth, a picture of toothpaste means putting toothpaste away, etc.).
- Keep kids focused on long-term goals by posting reminder pictures of coveted big rewards with the number of points/chips they cost in various locations. One mother posted a Six Flags amusement park ad on the wall where her son would see it in the morning when he awoke, on the refrigerator door, and in the garage (which he was responsible for cleaning). She pasted the number 1,000 on it to motivate her 11-year-old son to earn the 1,000 points he needed before the end of summer to take a friend to the park for a day. Lenny's mother posted Chicago Bulls insignia all over the house to remind her son that he needed 500 points to get the Bulls jersey he craved.
- Especially for older kids, money can be a motivating reward, but always put a limit on how many chips or points can be turned in for money each week so money is not the only reward the child purchases. Give the money earned by the child weekly as an allowance.
- Four- to seven-year-olds should be permitted to take their chips out of the bank to redeem them for rewards by handing them over to you. Performing this physical act becomes a ritual that only reinforces the incentive.
- Keep the unearned chips out of reach of your defiant child.

Some children simply find it too tempting to make unauthorized "deposits" into their own bank.

• This program is a new habit for you, too, so help yourself get into the routine by posting reminders to stop what you're doing every 20 or 30 minutes during this first week and check on your child to see if a reward is in order. Try setting your kitchen timer or watch alarm. Some parents put little stickers, such as smiley faces, around the house where they'll see them regularly—the refrigerator, the phone receiver, a mirror, a clock face, various doors, and so forth.

• What if you have more than one defiant child? One family with twins, both of whom had ADHD, bought two different sets of poker chips—one plain and one with a gold horse stamped on it—for the kids. That way neither twin was tempted to "borrow" chips from the other.

Trouble Spots and Stumbling Blocks

"What happens when someone else is in charge of our son? Will the program work if he gets chips only when we're around?"

In Chapters 10 and 11 I'll explain how you can use this and other techniques in the program when you're out in public or the child is at school. There are, of course, also times when your child is supervised by someone else at home. In our experience, children are not embarrassed by the system; on the contrary, they can be so enthusiastic and proud of their ability to earn points that they willingly share the experience. One couple reported that their concern about leaving their six-year-old son with a baby-sitter dissolved when they walked into the living room to say good-bye and found their son explaining the whole system to the baby-sitter, showing off how many chips he already had in his bank. The sitter, who had had her own problems with the boy in the past, was understandably enthusiastic about participating.

One caveat: Allow baby-sitters to get involved with the program only if they are responsible people in their late teens or adults and they care for the child often. Younger sitters and ones who don't see or know the child well will probably misinterpret the program and could counter the strides you make by treating it as a way to penalize rather than reward the child.

The same goes for grandparents. Unless they take care of your child as regular sitters, such as daily while you're at work, they should not be involved.

We recommend in such cases that the sitter or grandparent be given a notebook or steno pad to record various behaviors, both good and bad. Then, when you come home, you review it and dispense points or fines, respectively, as a consequence. This gives sitters and grandparents some authority—they can write things in "the book"—but the parents have the final say as to how many points are given or taken back.

"Our daughter listed a whole bunch of privileges that she hasn't 'bought' once this week. Does this mean the program isn't working?"

No, as long as she is showing interest in earning some of the rewards on the list and is willing to behave well to do so. The list of privileges always requires ongoing adjustments to make it as effective as it can be. Review the list periodically, say once a month, and make any changes your experience dictates. Cut privileges that are never or rarely redeemed and ask your child which new ones he or she might be interested in.

"I got carried away this week and put a bunch of jobs on the list that my child hasn't done at all. How should I react to that?"

As with privileges, you should hold a regular review of the jobs listed. Sometimes parents get so enthusiastic about the potential for improving their child's behavior that they include the whole laundry list of things they'd love to see the child accomplish, regardless of whether it is realistic to expect these achievements from the child. The best approach is to start with a great majority of jobs that you know your child can do but has trouble doing consistently. This way the child has a chance to earn points for doing these things and is motivated to try to do them more often to increase the earnings. If you're trying to discourage certain behaviors, such as interrupting you, make it possible for the child to earn points for small increments of time without interrupting. This way the child can see some success from not interrupting you even for 5 minutes and will be motivated by the chips earned to try to stretch it to 15 to triple the earnings.

"How long should I keep up this program? Will my child ever be able to do without it?"

I always find it interesting when parents want to discuss stopping a technique before it even begins. This may reflect lack of readiness for change. Some parents talk a good game, but when they actually have to do something to help their child, we see signs of low commitment. This can be one of them. But it can also mean, in cases of ADHD, that the parents don't really understand that ADHD is a developmental disability. If this child had a physical handicap that kept her in a wheelchair, no parent would say, "How long do I have to use the wheelchair with my child?" Likewise, parents of ADHD children need to understand that using artificial reward programs is almost a necessity for ADHD kids, given their motivational disability.

Please plan on keeping this program up for two months—the entire program plus a few weeks following the last step. In our experience, parents usually find themselves fading the program out somewhat naturally, perhaps because the child's behavior has improved a lot but also because parents begin to get lax and inconsistent over time. If this happens without any relapse in the child's behavior, just continue as you are. If for some reason you have a great desire to stop using the rewards program altogether, tell the child that you're going to try life without it for one or two days: The child will still have the daily privileges usually earned, but only if he or she is behaving well and complying with most of your requests. If the child's behavior remains as good as it was with the program in place, you can extend the trial period indefinitely. If behavior becomes a problem again, reinstate the program—pronto.

"Annie keeps asking for 'advances' on her chips because she doesn't have enough to watch a full hour of TV and 'really really has to see the new "Goosebumps" story.' I've caved in a couple of times but have a funny feeling this isn't getting us anywhere. What should I say next time she asks?"

Just explain very firmly that, as you told Annie when the program began, no chips will be awarded unless she behaves well in some specific way—either by complying with your first request that she do something or not do something, by doing a job with a particularly great attitude, or by doing something special that's not on the list. Only by holding back the privileges until she earns them will you help Annie learn that she must think ahead.

"It seems so cruel to charge my son for things he's always taken for granted as a member of this family. How can I explain this without making him feel like he's not as good as the rest of us?"

This is tough, I know. Remember, emphasize the positive, and stress when you introduce the program that its purpose is to reward all the great things your son has been doing. (Even if he doesn't do too many terrific things right now in your eyes, he'll be motivated to begin if you express this confidence in him.) If he tries to compare himself to a sibling, gently point out specific things that are a problem for him that his sibling doesn't have a problem with—getting dressed for school on time, avoiding hitting friends, doing a chore the first time he's asked, and so forth.

Depending on the age and mental capacity of your son, you can also try to explain the system in the larger social context: Privileges and rewards, just like most things we want in life, have to be earned by behaving well within our society. This applies to adults as well as to children. We all have to obey the law and follow rules and regulations, and we're expected to meet certain standards for social conduct, such as courtesy, respect, and kindness, if we want to be treated in kind. The harder the child works on this program, the greater the rewards, in the same way that additional work on the job might get us a bonus or a promotion. The more you can give your child real experiences of your own as examples, the more credible your explanations will be. You can also explain that this poker chip/point system is really just like our monetary system: We work to earn a salary or wages, which we use to provide the things we want and need in life.

"Doesn't this system deliver some bad messages, like bribery is OK, and it's OK to reward one kid for something but not another?"

Some children, like your defiant child, simply need this kind of incentive where others do not. Without this device, at least for the time being, your child will remain disabled. Wouldn't you rather give your child this prosthetic device so he has a chance of behaving like the other kids? However, it might help to remember that even so-called normal children respond better to being rewarded than to not being rewarded. A seven-year-old girl who makes her bed without being asked is likely to get pretty lax if no one notices, but when her bedtime is pushed back an extra 15 minutes because "she's so grown-up," she starts clearing the table after dinner without being asked as well. "Normal" children are in fact rewarded for good behavior all the time; it's just that there usually is no formal system in place like this one. Finally, remember that bribery means paying someone to do something wrong. As you should know if you've ever held a paying job or won an award for volunteer work, there's nothing wrong with being rewarded for doing something right.

"My child has turned into an angel overnight after just a week at Step 3. Can this possibly last?"

You can expect the gains to be sustained, but perhaps not with this level of devotion or motivation. We have found that there is about a two- to three-week honeymoon period with a new chip program where the child is unusually motivated to work. Once the program becomes routine and the novelty wears off a bit, so does some of the child's motivation to work. Children don't quit working; they just back off a bit on their ambition. That's why the fines kick in a week or two later, in Step 4.

"My husband doesn't want to get involved in the reward program—he says he really doesn't need to since I'm handling it all day long. Is it OK for me to do this alone?"

No, it's not. Mothers often play the larger role in this step if they're the ones staying at home with the kids, but you're not going to get the consistency in child management that you need unless both of you use the system whenever you're around. Help your husband out by showing him a few of the child's behaviors that he can easily recognize and reward in the evenings—maybe not interrupting dinner conversations or taking the dog out for an evening walk without being asked. Once he gets the hang of it, he'll be sucked into success just like you are.

"My child simply refused to participate when I introduced the program, despite the fact that I put a lot of enthusiasm into presenting it positively. What can I do?"

This is a rare reaction, but it is seen among highly oppositional children sometimes. When it does happen, I tell parents to go ahead with it on their own. List the fun things that your child enjoys as privileges every day and simply withhold them if the child doesn't earn any points. Within a few days, the child is likely to begin cooperating, even if grudgingly.

"Wow, this sounds time-consuming. How can I fit this in on top of holding special times and remembering to praise and monitor my child all the time? What about the rest of my life?"

Yes, this will take some time to get used to during the first week, but it will become a regular habit and thus not too onerous soon thereafter, especially because your child will be so motivated to help. (Believe me, your son or daughter will be happy to go fetch the "bank book" or chip bank for deposits or withdrawals!) If you get tired or discouraged this week, please remember that I'm asking you to spend a mere two months undoing possibly a lifetime of defiance—it's time very well spent.

"This program already seems to be helping my son. Can I try it with my other kids?"

As I said earlier, even nondefiant children improve their behavior when they're on a reward system like this. Still, whether you use it for all your kids is an individual decision. Certainly, the more different "bank accounts" you have to keep track of, the more time-consuming the program is. However, it may be worth it if keeping privilege granting and job monitoring consistent and predictable is a priority in your house. Brothers and sisters often ask parents if they can participate once they see how much easier it is to figure out the circumstances under which they'll be allowed to pursue certain desirable activities.

"How do I know exactly how well the program is working?"

You should see more consistency in the child's ability to behave well over the course of a day. Systematically providing the reward of points or chips that can be turned in for an interesting variety of privileges prevents the child's motivation to comply from fluctuating as much as it has in the past. Because these rewards and the privileges they can buy are more powerful than praise and attention alone, you can expect your child to progress more rapidly now, with compliance increasing in much more noticeable increments. Also, you should feel more relaxed and confident if this program is working. Taking a more organized, more systematic, and fairer approach to managing the child's behavior means fewer nasty surprises for everyone. You don't have to listen to "That's not fair!" arguments if you're sticking to the program, and your child doesn't have to live with the uncertainty of wondering when you're going to bestow a special privilege just because you happen to be in a good mood—or withhold it because you're in a bad mood. Finally, the need to hand out tokens and watch for good behavior forces you to pay still more attention to your child, and in turn your child will be seeking your attention to get those rewards. You can't help getting closer, and that's the way the parent–child relationship is meant to be.

If this is a fair description of what you're experiencing, you're more than halfway home. The next chapter will flesh out your skills by giving you another powerful tool, this one for getting over the rough spots that are bound to appear in even the smoothest path.

This approach to child management is important for a number of reasons: It helps to counter the lack of motivation that some defiant kids have, especially in cases of ADHD. It makes the rules and the consequences in the home very clear, fair, and certain or predictable, putting an end to indiscriminate parenting. It helps to reorganize family transactions so that they are more positive and parents are more attentive to child prosocial and work-related behavior. It teaches an important work ethic that is the foundation of this country—you get what you work for, and there is no free lunch. It makes kids feel good to know that their work in the family is appreciated. Finally, it is one of the most powerful techniques for changing child behavior in this program.

CHAPTER 8

Step 4:
Use Mild Discipline—
Time-Out and More

Before . . .

"I don't care if I get any points today!" Maya shouted.

Joy's jaw dropped as she turned to stare at her nine-year-old daughter. The girl she'd been living with for the last week had generally been a pleasure to be around—agreeable, relatively good-natured, and very enthusiastic about earning points toward everything from TV time to special outings with family or friends. Who was this girl?

"Well, then," Joy replied hesitantly, "I guess you're not going to get much TV time today . . ."

"I said I don't care!" Maya shouted back.

As Maya trudged out of the room, Joy tried to figure out what had gone wrong. Had she asked Maya to do something unusual? No, her daughter had happily packed up her own backpack every morning since she'd been getting points for doing it. Had she expected too much of Maya this morning? No, it had been pretty much before-school business as usual. Had she asked too "nicely," giving her daughter an easy out? No, she hadn't deviated from her new habit of simple statements: "Maya, it's time to pack your backpack for school." Maybe her daughter had just gotten up on the wrong side of the bed. Joy packed her daughter's bag and hoped that things would be better after school.

They weren't. At 3:30 sharp, Maya came barreling through the front door, threw her pack on the floor, tossed her coat onto the bannister, and charged into her room, leaving the door gaping open. A gust of cold air brought Joy rushing out of her home office to investigate.

"Maya! Get back here and close the door, pick up your stuff . . . and you could at least say hello to your mother!"

"I'm busy!" Maya yelled back.

The rest of the day was a downward spiral of ignored requests, defied commands, and backtalk alternating with glum silence.

"What a nightmare," Joy complained to a friend on the phone once Maya was finally in bed. "We ended up screaming at each other just like in the 'old days,' and finally, when she told me she could go to bed whenever she felt like it because I was always too busy working to notice anyway, I told her she was grounded for a month. I immediately apologized, and she gave me that sly look that said we both knew I never would have stuck to it. I feel like a fool—I must have undone everything we've been working on. How could I let her get to me like that?"

After . . .

I don't care if I get any points today!" Maya shouted.

Joy's jaw dropped as she turned to stare at her nine-year-old daughter. The scowl on her daughter's face and her hands-on-hips stance delivered a silent "I dare you" message to her mother.

Joy stifled a retort, then looked her daughter directly in the eyes and said firmly, "It's time to get ready for school. Start packing your backpack now."

"No!" shouted her daughter.

"OK," countered Joy, "then I'm subtracting five points from your bank book."

"That's not fair," her daughter yelled and tried to grab the notebook from her mother's hands.

"Stop that shouting right now," Joy said, "and start packing your back-pack. Five . . . four . . . three. . . ."

Maya continued shouting "No fair!" and when Joy got down to "one," she said, "If you don't pack that backpack right now, you're going to sit in that chair." She pointed to the lone chair sitting in a corner of the family room. "Five . . . four . . . three . . . two . . . one."

Joy took her daughter by the arm and drew her over to the chair, setting her firmly into it. "You're going to stay there until I say you can leave."

Joy walked into the kitchen, where she started packing the kids' lunches. She could see Maya from where she worked but ignored her daughter's non-stop complaining. After 10 minutes, she went back to the chair and said, "You can't leave the chair until you're quiet. I'm not coming back until then."

After a few minutes, Maya's complaints had reduced to whimpers and then finally to silence. Joy returned to the chair and said, "Are you ready to pack your backpack?"

"Yes," Maya answered quietly.

"OK, go do it—it's almost time for the bus."

Maya got up and packed her backpack quickly. Joy watched and said, "I like it when you do as I ask."

On her way out the door a few minutes later, Maya turned and said softly, "Sorry, Mom."

The home token system you set up in Step 3 is a compelling tool, but it's not omnipotent. Most children, even those who seem completely transformed by working for rewards, will fall back into bad behavior at some point, for some reason. Other children emerge from Step 3 with the motivation to cooperate in many areas of their life, but some specific problems will persist. Either way, you'll need another way to nudge them back on track.

Joy in the "before" scenario illustrates how easy it is to be lulled into a false sense of security by the radical positive changes that the point system can bring about. When their defiant child seems transformed by the incentive of rewards, parents hope and pray that the change will endure, and it often does. We have found, however, that the honeymoon usually doesn't last more than three or four weeks. Beyond that period, you'd best brace yourself for at least occasional noncompliance. Remember, you haven't changed your child's inner wiring, and even your best efforts to avoid overloading the circuits will sometimes be thwarted. If you're not prepared for these relapses, old habits of interacting can rush to the surface and drag you and your child down into the maelstrom of push-and-pull conflict so fast that your rebuilt relationship will seem to crumble around you.

Lingering behavior problems, from having trouble getting along with other kids to failing to finish chores, can have a more insidious effect. Your inability to make inroads in certain areas can make you feel helpless, and feelings of helplessness have a way of overshadowing the confidence you should get from your successes over time. With some children, frankly, you may not be able to resolve every single behavior problem. You can, however, take satisfaction in knowing you're doing everything you can to help your child get past these snags. For that reason it's important to take this additional step and add disincentives to boost the incentives you're already offering.

In addition to giving your incentive efforts a boost, the punishment techniques presented in this chapter will give the boot to any vestiges of your old child management methods. As you know, punishment has been strictly omitted from the lessons of Steps 1–3, but you've been given permission to use your usual punishment when you simply had to put a stop to extremely bad behavior. Now we're going to replace those old ways of penalizing your child—measures that may have stopped the immediate offense but encouraged a repeat performance—with two mild methods that will make you a fair and consistent disciplinarian. I can't remind you too often how important predictability is to building trust and cooperation. So think of these new punishment tools as the final brick in your renovated relationship with your child—the replacement of one last shaky building block with a truly solid support.

First, though, thoroughly inspect your foundation. You should not even consider adopting the punishment methods in Step 4 until you have laid down a dependable base of praise, attention, and rewards. If your child still behaves poorly in many circumstances, it may be that your positive reinforcement skills need work, not that you need to introduce punishment. If you've seen very little or no improvement in your child's behavior with Step 3, examine the approach you've taken. In one family I counseled, homemaker Mom adopted the program correctly, but lawyer Dad was home so seldom that he often gave chips away for nothing. Or he waited until bedtime and then gave chips to the child for having such a "great day" according to Mom. This indiscriminate use of chips severely undermined the program. The kid had plenty of chips to spend but was not really earning some of them, thanks to Dad. At that point we had a pretty blunt talk about the fact that the child's current behavior was the best predictor of future delinquency. When I pointed out that his son was eventually going to need a good lawyer of his own if both parents did not commit to the program, the boy's father agreed to give it a more concerted effort, and the boy's behavior improved.

Your ultimate goal is never to impose punishment until you've pulled all the other arrows out of your quiver. So this is a good time to get used to asking why your child is misbehaving, as Joy did in the "before" scenario. By focusing on the positive and getting back into your child's corner, you have made it possible to stay calm in interactions with your child. Now it's not so easy to push your buttons, and you have a chance in any encounter to ask yourself why the child is misbehaving before you plunge into emotional overreaction. There's never any harm in rushing into praise, but the same cannot be said for punishment. So try to get in the habit of doing a quick survey of the circumstances before you resort to punishment. These are the kinds of questions you should learn to ask yourself reflexively:

- *Am I making my commands effectively, as learned in Step 2?*
- *Am I demonstrating my willingness to follow through, or am I inviting my child to test me?*
- *Have I paid attention to the need for new and different rewards and privileges as my child grows and changes?* When in doubt, take another look at the list of things your child likes that you wrote up at the end of Chapter 3. Do you think it has changed? If you're not sure, ask your child to review it with you.
- *Am I remaining sensitive to my child's characteristics and personal challenges in our interactions?* If you need some help here, periodically review the questionnaires you filled out on pages 29–33 of Chapter 2.
- *Are my own personal problems or traits harming how I act with my child?* Review the questionnaires on pages 35–36 and 45–46 of Chapter 2 to remind yourself of the influences in your own life that could be seeping into your encounters with your child.
- *Could any new external factors be causing my child to behave badly?* Besides your own personality and problems identified in Chapter 2, look for problems at school, in the neighborhood, or with your child's physical health or development that might be stressful.

Obviously, some questions will have to be put off until you have time to do the necessary exploration and introspection. The idea is not to paralyze yourself but to be aware of answers you need to seek at a later time. Never punish a child without trying to understand why the child misbehaved, but never get so lost in thought *at the time of the misbehavior* that you fail to do something about it.

That said, the greatest challenge in Step 4 is not to overcome a tendency to punish your child too much but to stick with your new approach to discipline. At first, your child will not understand that you are replacing indiscriminate discipline with a reasonable and predictable system. All your son or daughter will see is that you're introducing something new and unpleasant—compared to the undeniably pleasant praise, attention, and rewards that you've been giving out over the last few weeks. Not surprisingly, many children feel betrayed and tricked when you start taking points away or isolating them from family and fun for misbehavior. Unfortunately, many instinctively respond the way they did to your old punishment techniques—with worse behavior.

Because of the negative reactions your child is likely to have, this will be the most difficult week of the program. Children often respond to the first instances of punishment by throwing temper tantrums—sometimes very long ones—and you'll need to marshal all your inner forces to resist giving in. Some kids will try to hit you where it hurts—in the heart—by telling you that you're horrible and that they don't love you anymore. There are several ways that you can gird yourself for this onslaught.

1. Understand that extreme negative reactions like these are usually a solid indication that the methods will eventually have the effect you're after—they'll discourage your child from pursuing the punished behavior.

2. Remind yourself of your child's positive attributes. You listed them at the end of Chapter 3, and remembering what you like and admire about your child now will help you withstand the histrionics and abuse later.

3. Remind yourself of what you've accomplished so far. Even if it's not all you hoped for, you've seen progress. Take out a sheet of paper and quickly jot a list under the heading "How Life with [child's name] Has Improved." I hope this list will motivate you to go on.

4. Remind yourself of why you're taking the time and effort to go through this program: You love your child and want the best for him or her. Keeping this thought in mind may help when the little darling accuses you of being "a mean old monster" who just doesn't care.

5. Draw up a simple plan for staying relaxed and renewed. You're going to need to devote a lot of energy to the program this week, and you'll need to replenish it. Plan a dinner out once or twice if you can. Schedule a hot bath with a good book for the quiet time after your child is in bed. Remember to exercise. Figure out what makes *you* feel good when you're under stress and do what you can to get it.

6. Bear in mind that your child, knowingly or not, has become a great actor. She believes that if she displays all of her anger and upset with you, you will cave in once again and relent on your punishment. Tell yourself you are not going to be conned this time around. You stand firm for your principles and you care about the long-term interests of the child. Give in, and you teach your child, once again, that displays of anger and tantrums make others succumb to what she wants. Is that what you really want to teach? Sometimes you must expose your child to things that upset her for her own long-term best interest. Remember when you first took your child for her inoculations at the pediatrician? You were having her stuck with needles, and she cried over it and hated it. But you did it anyway because you knew it was in her best interest in the long run, despite her unhappiness with you at the moment. Your time-out program is exactly the same, and your attitude toward it should be exactly the same as well. Good parents look out for the long-term best interests of their children and not just their short-term "feel good" interests.

7. Remember the positive reinforcement! It may take all the stamina you have, but the fact that your child just threw a two-hour tantrum should not alter your usual game plan of praise and attention. Special time has never been more important—don't give up on it now!

Reintroducing Punishment

For this week, the goal is to gradually reintroduce punishment in a way that is firm and consistent. Here is what you'll do:

1. Begin deducting points or chips when the child fails to do a task that is normally rewarded in the home token system.
2. Write up a short list of social misbehaviors for which the child is to be fined as well.
3. Learn how to use time-out.
4. Choose one or two behavior problems for which you'll use time-out this week.
5. Follow the rule "Fine twice, then isolate." For any infraction that is repeated or continued, despite the first fine you impose, fine the child only once more before using time-out.

Method 1: Fines for Misbehavior

Children who have been racking up chips or points via the home token system will naturally be discouraged or even outraged by being fined for misbehavior, but once you have seen solid benefits from rewarding the child for compliance, you're ready to start imposing consequences for noncompliance. For failure to comply with a command or chore, simply subtract the number of points the child would have received for complying. (If the child gets five points for making his bed in the morning, not making the bed would mean missing out on the five points that could have been earned and also losing five points already earned.)

If you are not already rewarding the child specifically for *not* throwing a tantrum, teasing her brother, lying to Mom and Dad, or breaking some household rule, how much do you fine the child for committing these "crimes"? Essentially, the more extreme the misbehavior, the greater the penalty you should impose. Serious offenses should result in a loss of as much as one-third or more of the child's typical daily income. Taking away everything the child has earned that day would be too severe, but fines that amount to only 5 to 10% of daily income may be too light. About 25 to 30% of daily income should be sufficient to make the point without bankrupting the child. However, if the same misbehavior is repeated that day, increase the next fine by 10%. To avoid a punishment spiral (see page 161), remember the "Fine twice, then isolate" rule.

Method 2: Time-Out for Acting Out

From now on, you're going to start issuing commands only if you're willing to impose a consequence for not complying with them. Because so many defiant children would spend their entire day sitting in the time-out chair if every type of offense were punished this way, though, your job this week is to use time-out with only one or two areas that are a common problem for your child. If your child still has many behavior problems, you might choose one often uncompleted chore and one social problem to target this week. So the child might get time-out for not taking any dishes used into the kitchen and for interrupting conversations at the dinner table. If the child has one big, constant problem area, such as not cleaning up after herself, focus solely on that this week. If you're the lucky parent of a child whose problems have been resolved almost entirely by Step 3's home token system, just wait; your day will come, usually within another week or two. No child is perfect, and yours is bound to try some of his old behaviors with you once the glow of the token system wears off a bit more. Just be ready to use your penalties when this happens.

Time-out can be used with all children aged 2 through 12 but is probably most effective with ages 2 through 10.

To prepare for this step, find a straight-backed chair such as a dinette chair or an old-fashioned wooden classroom chair and place it in a spot where you'll be able to see the child while going about your normal household routine. Effective spots are in the foyer, in the middle of a hallway, or in a corner of the dining room or kitchen. Make sure the chair is far enough from the walls to prevent the child from kicking them and that the child won't be able to reach anything to play or fiddle with while in the chair. Be sure to choose a spot where you can leave this chair for at least two weeks as a reminder to the child of the consequences for misbehaving. (This usually means making sure it's not in the way of other family members.)

For this week, whenever you have to ask your child to do something in the designated category, follow these steps:

1. Give the command (such as "Tyler, put your dirty clothes in the laundry hamper"), following the guidelines for effective commands that you learned in Step 3. Out loud, begin to count backward, starting with five and counting at intervals of about one second for each number.

2. If your child does not start to obey by the time you reach one—after about five seconds have passed—make direct eye contact with your child and use body language that tells your child you mean business: Adopt a firmer posture and stance, point your finger at the child, and say more loudly than when you gave the original command, "If you don't do as I say, you're going to sit in that chair!" ("If you don't put your clothes in the hamper as I asked, you're going to sit in that chair!") Then point to the time-out chair you've set up.

3. Now start counting down from five again. If you reach one again, say, "You didn't do as I said, so you are going to the chair." ("You didn't put your clothes in the hamper as I asked, so you are going to the chair.")

4. Then firmly take the child by the wrist or upper arm and escort him or her to the chair. Now say, "You sit there until I say you can get up," and make sure your voice is loud and firm so the child will know you mean it.

5. Leave the child in the chair for one or two minutes for each year of the child's age—one minute for lesser infractions, two minutes for more severe violations. While the child is in time-out, go about your business where you can keep an eye on the child, but don't get involved in any discussions or arguments. The child probably will not sit there quietly, but you should ignore anything he or she says.

6. When the time is up, go over to the child and say, if he or she is making noise, "I'm not coming back to the chair until you're quiet." Then go back to what you were doing and don't return until the child has been quiet for about 30 seconds.

7. Once the child has been quiet for a moment, go back to the chair and ask if the child is ready to do what you asked. ("Are you ready to put your clothes in the hamper, Tyler?" or, when the child has done something wrong that cannot be undone, "Are you ready to promise never to hit Charles again?")

If the child says yes, make sure he actually follows through. (If the child later hits Billy again, immediately take him back to the time-out chair, without a command or warning.) If he does not, take him right back to the chair and start over.

If the child says no, start over, with "All right, then you stay there until I say you can get up!" Repeat this as many times as you have to until the child does what you asked.

8. Once the child has done what you ask, say in a neutral tone of voice, "I like it when you do what I ask." Don't gush over the child's compliance or give any rewards for it. Do, however, watch the child carefully so you'll catch the next significant good behavior. When you do, be sure to reward it as you learned to do in Steps 2 and 3. This maintains the precarious balance of positive and negative and also demonstrates that you don't dislike your son or daughter but used time-out only as punishment for misbehavior.

Exceptions to the Procedure

Certain circumstances may call for a slightly varied procedure.

- *For violations of household rules:* The child should be sent to time-out without a command or warning anytime he or she breaks a household rule that is clearly understood. These rules might include "no hitting," "no stealing," "no playing with knives," "no using the stove," "no snacking without permission." To be absolutely clear about this, post a list of the rules you know are often broken—someplace like the refrigerator door where the list will be highly visible—and tell the child at the beginning of this week that if she breaks any of the rules she'll be sent to time-out without any warning.

- *For longer tasks:* If your child has a longer task to perform, such as completing a homework assignment, it's just as important that the job be finished as that it be started. So, instead of giving a command and warning as detailed above, tell the child that he has a certain amount of time to complete the job and that if he doesn't do that he'll be sent to time-out. Then set the timer to avoid any argument about how much time really went by.

- *For repeated offenses:* If the child has been released from time-out upon the promise not to repeat the misbehavior (such as hitting Billy, above), no command or warning should be given before returning the child to time-out if he does repeat the misbehavior.

Dos and Don'ts

- **Don't** begin Step 4 at a time when special family activities that would distract you from this program are scheduled. If you can't put off the special event because it's something like a wedding or a visit from out-of-town friends or relatives, stay at Step 3 for another week, until you have the time to concentrate on your efforts here.

- **Don't** continue counting out loud after a few weeks of using time-out. Otherwise, you'll teach your child to obey only those commands followed by a countdown.

- **Don't** overdo it when adopting a firm tone and stance. How tough you'll need to appear depends on how defiant your child tends to be and the body language you usually use. The important thing is to escalate the firmness of your message if your child does not comply right away. This may mean getting up from your chair to deliver your second command or warning, or it may mean firmly planting your feet on the floor and standing up straighter rather than slouching with hand on hip as you may have done while giving the initial command. You usually don't have to be theatrical to get your point across. Remember, once you use a particular tone that says "I mean it," anything less won't be taken seriously.

- **Don't** put the time-out chair in a closet, a stairway into a basement, or a bathroom. Many children are afraid of the dark, and your goal is not to torture them with those fears but only to remove them from ongoing rewarding activities. The bathroom is not permitted because it is dangerous. It's tough to keep an eye on the child from other parts of the house, so use a place that is easily observable and safe.

- **Don't** allow brothers, sisters, or other people in the house to speak to the child while he or she is in the time-out chair.

- **Don't** apologize for having had to punish the child once the time-out is up and the child has agreed to comply.

Forewarned Is Forearmed

Again, most children will react negatively—some in the extreme—to your adding token penalties and time-out to your reinforcement arsenal. Anticipate the worst and profit by the experiences of parents who have been through it already.

When a Child Fights the Fine . . .

• Be on the lookout for a phenomenon I call the "punishment spiral": When you first fine your child, he may very well throw a tantrum, swear at you, or strike out at someone or something in rage. This is obviously unacceptable behavior, so you may be tempted to respond by fining the child again. This leads to further resistance by your child and another fine from you. Eventually the child ends up with so many deductions that he can't hope to make them up with positive behavior and therefore can't hope to earn any privileges. As you can undoubtedly guess, the child who ends up in this situation loses motivation to earn points pretty fast. The solution: If your child reacts inappropriately to being fined, fine her only one more time. Then send the child to time-out.

• Some children get so angry that points are being deducted from their balance without being spent on privileges that they decide to reject the whole system. The key is to persist. One boy flushed the checkbook register being used to keep track of his points down the toilet the first time his parents fined him for misbehavior. His parents started the whole system again with a new register, and they did the same thing when he flushed the second one. Eventually the boy realized his parents weren't going to be headed off so easily, and he gave in.

• Some children react to the announcement that points or chips will be deducted with "Go ahead—I don't care." Don't be put off if your child says this. It's almost always a smoke screen. If you know for a fact that your child does care about the privilege that will be lost along with the loss of points, you can hear the child's true meaning: "I don't like what you're doing and I want you to stop."

When the Child Tries to Get Out of Time-Out . . .

• The first escape route the child is likely to try is to agree to comply with your request as soon as you've told him or her to sit in the chair now. Don't allow it. Once you've counted down from five twice, it's too late, and the child must pay the consequences.

• If the child physically resists being taken to the time-out chair, you can use *slight* force to make sure the child gets there—meaning picking the child up bodily or taking hold of both of his arms to lead him to the chair, *not* using brute force or in any way hurting the child. If your child is physically aggressive, you need to take extra care—see the box on page 165.

• An all-out tantrum on the way to or in the chair is not uncommon. Again, stick to your guns and have the child stay in the chair until he can be quiet for at least 30 seconds—even if this means sitting in the chair for 1 or 2 hours. Many parents can attest to the fact that it usually takes only one such marathon before children realize that you can hold out longer than they can. Once they realize that quieting down cuts down on the time served in the chair, they quickly shorten their stays there.

One family had their son serve his time-out in his bedroom, where, the first time around, they heard him kicking his walls and throwing things on the floor. Their solution was to help him cool off by sitting on the bed and holding him. When he calmed down, he had to serve his time-out.

• Many children simply take it on the lam—they leave the chair at the first opportunity. In this case, you have several options. The most common route is to move the child to the bedroom, like this: The first time the child tries to leave the chair, place her back in it and say firmly, "If you get out of that chair again, I'm going to send you to your bed!" Use the same firm stance and loud voice as when warning the child to comply before giving a time-out. If the child moves again, send her to her room, put her on the bed, and tell her she has to sit there until you say she can leave. Be sure that no major toys or other forms of entertainment (TV, stereo, etc.) are in the bedroom. If the child tries to leave the bedroom, close and lock the door. The child has to complete the time-out as described above.

A few parents have told me they are afraid that using the child's bedroom for time-out will cause their child sleep problems because it confuses the bedroom with punishment. I have never seen that happen, and there is no research to back it up. Other parents have expressed fear that their child will destroy the room. I tell these parents that any destruction is reparable, but they get only one shot at raising a child properly. Many parents actually prefer the child's room to the chair method, but if you don't, you can try one of the following alternatives: (1) subtract points or chips for leaving the chair; (2) for older children, deny the child a highly valued privilege that would have been granted later in the day (such as watching a football playoff game); (3) add five minutes to the time-out interval for each attempt to leave the chair (which can go on ad infinitum and also encourage game playing by the child). If none of these methods works, you need to see a professional.

   • Many kids will try to push your buttons, complaining "I hate you," "You don't love me," or variations on the old favorite, "You're so mean." Although these accusations may sound easy to fend off on paper, they can really get to you when they're coming from the mouth of your beloved child and when you take them at face value. The first thing you should *not* do is encourage this abuse by taking the time to respond that of course you love your little boy or girl. This just says "Please do this again if you want my attention." The first thing you *should* do is take whatever measure you need to remove yourself emotionally from the assault. One mother of a son who would yell, "You're a terrible mother" and "No one else has a mother as mean as you" decided she had to imagine that she was a diplomat listening to a foreign-language speech through the headphones that the UN representatives use to hear translations. Through these imaginary headphones, she would "interpret" her son's message: "I don't like being in time-out, and I want you to let me out." This tactic didn't stop her son's verbal attacks, but it lifted the awful emotional burden imposed on his mother.
   • Some children will decide that if they can't dissuade you from imposing time-out, they'll turn the punishment on you and do everything they can to annoy you by tipping, rocking, or moving the chair. There's only one way to handle this: Tell your child that if the chair is moving, it's the same thing as trying to leave it. Then apply the same consequences as for leaving the chair.
   • Then there's the old "I have to go to the bathroom" ploy. In 20 years of using this program with thousands of children, I've heard of only two who have followed through on a threat to wet their pants if they couldn't get up and go to the bathroom, and those children clear-

ly did so intentionally to defy their parents. These two had smart parents who kept them in the chair until their time was up, then had them clean up the area and change their clothes. The wrong response is to cave in; not only will your child resort to this trick again and again, but you'll find it awfully difficult to get the child back in the chair once he or she has gone to the bathroom. One mother who called the bluff of a six-year-old who said she would wet her pants found the little girl didn't wet her pants—and never used that excuse again. When in doubt, remember that even for a 10-year-old the maximum time spent in the chair if the child agrees to comply after the minimum "sentence" is 20 minutes, and I don't know of any 10-year-olds who can't wait that long to use the bathroom.

• "I don't feel good" is another common ploy. Kids who have been throwing a tantrum may mean it when they complain of a sore throat, but it will pass. Others claim to have a headache or stomachache and can alarm their parents by claiming they will throw up if they have to stay in the chair. Unless the child actually has shown the symptoms of illness earlier in the day when time-out was not an issue, don't fall for this. The only child I've ever known who vomited after making this threat stuck his finger down his throat in an act of deliberate defiance and had to clean up after himself.

• "I'm tired" is a complaint heard typically when time-out is used near bedtime. Should you pay attention? Probably not. Although I discourage parents from punishing resistance to bedtime with time-out during this first week because this problem often goes away when the success of time-out generalizes to other behavior problems, I don't think you should hesitate to keep a child up a few minutes past bedtime to enforce a time-out. Will this just give the child what so many of them want? It's unlikely that any child will find sitting in a chair by himself with nothing to do a triumph in terms of staying up past bedtime. On the other hand, if a time-out at bedtime means the child isn't missing anything but sleep, the time may have to be extended to the full two minutes per year of age to make it effective.

• Few parents can hold out against a child's claims of hunger, and many kids will hook you with this one while in time-out. Denying children food has too many Dickensian overtones for most of us, but try to keep in mind that your child is not going to waste away if she misses one snack or even a meal. If the child is sent to time-out during a meal, don't make any efforts to give the child a meal after the time-out is served. If the time-out is up before your family has finished its meal, the child can rejoin the family while they're eating, but the meal should not be extended to accommodate the defiant child. Remember, missing out on activities—including eating—while in time-out will lose its teeth as punishment if you then compensate for that loss afterward.

• Believe it or not, some children try to wrest control back from their parents by actually refusing to leave time-out once the time is up. What they're saying, in essence, is "*I'll* tell you when I want to leave this chair." The only thing to do is turn it back on them: Say that because the child has refused to do what you asked—to leave the chair—the child will have to start the time-out all over again and will stay in the chair until *you* say the child can leave.

WHEN A CHILD GETS PHYSICAL . . .

If your child has violent tendencies and is old enough to be a significant danger to you, he or she may very well have conduct disorder and should be treated professionally. See the Appendix at the end of the book (page 225) to get an idea of whether you should be concerned about the presence of CD in your child.

If your child tends toward physical aggression but is young and small, you may still feel uneasy about using time-out. In my experience, any such threats are always made to the mother, so the best approach this week is to use time-out only when the father is at home. There's a very good chance that your child will cooperate with you out of fear that the father will also get involved if the child does not go along with the punishment. If so, tell your child that this time-out period will be reduced by half because the child cooperated. Keep this up for the first week, then if all goes well, try using time-out once when the child's father is not at home. There's a good chance the child's cooperation will now extend to times when you are home alone together and you can proceed this way. If not, you'll have to seek professional help (see Chapter 3).

Trouble Spots
and Stumbling Blocks

"Why should I try this? Time-out is nothing new—I've tried it and it doesn't work."

Chances are the approach you tried was not the same as this one. Here is where your method probably differed from mine (and why it did not succeed):

- You probably used time-out as a last-resort punishment, when you were already furious, rather than systematically. This meant you had already repeated your commands several times, and the punishment therefore was not imposed immediately following noncompliance; you were so angry that you probably overdid the time period for the punishment; and you used the punishment indiscriminately.
- You probably left the punishment in the control of the child, making a statement that is painfully familiar to many of us: "Stay in your room until you're ready to behave!" Who's the parent here? *You* decide if and when the child is ready to leave the room.
- You may have set an arbitrary time-out period—say, 5 minutes—that you used regardless of the child's age or the severity of the problem. If you used 5 minutes for a 10-year-old, the punishment would have little effect. If you used 20 minutes for a 4-year-old or for a child of any age for a minor offense, you were shooting yourself in the foot.
- You may have caved in to pleas for mercy. If you let the child off the hook because he promised to comply as you were taking him to the chair or sending him to his room, time-out has not been a tool but an empty threat.

"How do I handle the things my child does wrong that we haven't targeted for time-out this week?"

You always have the alternative of fining the child for other misbehavior. If the child is acting out to an extreme, you can also make an exception and combine the two punishments.

"Our daughter's worst behavior is with her brother and sister—she never seems to stop bugging them. If we decide to use time-out for that problem this week, she'll be in the chair all day! But it really is her main problem, so what can we do?"

Try breaking down the problem into more narrowly defined violations. One family had a similar problem and wanted to establish the rule "Be nice to your sister" so they could punish the little boy whenever he wasn't "nice." I suggested that they replace that broad rule with "no hitting" and "no name calling." That way they would punish only the specific misbehaviors of hitting and name calling, and they could balance the punishment with positive reinforcement by giving praise or a bonus chip whenever their son played nicely or at least neutrally around his sister.

"One problem we've always had with Luke is that he claims not to have understood the rules. Any advice on keeping that from getting in our way with time-out and penalties?"

My best suggestion is to take a little time to be sure your expectations are understood. Again, post a list of rules that will be punished if violated. If your child can't read, use pictures as reminders. One mother wanted to be able to fine her son for violating the rule "No backtalk" but she was worried about whether he understood what that meant. So she spent a whole week saying, "That's what I mean by backtalk" whenever he was fresh to her and adding, "Starting next Tuesday you will lose 10 chips for that." She never heard a word of complaint about the fines once she began imposing them.

"My son lies all the time, and he's gotten very good at covering it up or denying it. How can I punish him if I'm not sure he's done anything wrong?"

You have to trust your own judgment and stand firm. One father who had the same concern decided to think of himself as his son's judge and jury. When he thought his son had lied to him or his mother, he would weigh the evidence and hand down a sentence, accepting the fact that he had not actually witnessed the "crime."

"I'd like to deal with my daughter's bad habit of tattling on her brothers, but I also know my sons and want to make sure she does tell me if anything dangerous is going on. How can I explain the difference to her?"

Many parents have the same complaint about their children, and this is a tricky issue. I counseled one couple who came up with a great solution: They told their son and daughter that before either of them came to the parents with a complaint about the other, they needed to think like a doctor who had a patient with a headache. Was the problem the kind that could be handled with the advice "Take two aspirin and call me in the morning?" or one that called for "We better get you to the hospital and take an X ray"? The kids were told that only the latter should be reported to the parents.

"What if slight physical force isn't enough to get my child into the chair?"

Do *not* use further physical force. Instead, fine the child a sizable fine—say 50% of his typical daily income—tell the child he is grounded for the day (no leaving the house, no playing with electronic devices, no phone calls with friends), then state that the grounding will be lifted once the child voluntarily goes to the chair and serves the time-out. The fine, however, stays in effect.

Remember, if you've tried all the provisions in this chapter and are still having problems with time-out, you should seek professional advice immediately.

"What do I do if my child commits one of the violations we've targeted for time-out while a visitor is in the house?"

Go ahead with the punishment. I know it may be embarrassing to you or the child, but if the child gets the message that all bets are off when outsiders are around, you can bet there will be lots of misbehavior when you least want to see it. Just calmly apologize to your guest and proceed as you would do without visitors. If the guest is a neighborhood child, just ask the child to leave.

"Our biggest problems with Julie are in stores and at church. We can't carry a chair around with us, so what can we do?"

Actually, there are effective ways to adapt time-out for use in public (covered in Chapter 10), but it's important to limit your use of time-out to the home for now. First of all, it's best to get one system—the at-home method—down solidly before moving on to variations. Second, you need to be confident enough in the method that you won't be too easily thrown by the reactions of strangers who witness your use of time-out in public. Third, there's a very good chance that time-out at home will be so effective with your child that the child's behavior overall will improve, including in public. Within just a few weeks, you may find you don't need it in public anymore.

"I'm exhausted and depressed—this feels like the worst week of my life and I'm ready to give up. What am I doing wrong?"

You're not doing anything wrong, and you're not alone in the way you feel. Most parents greatly dislike disciplining their children. It takes time and effort, it is not fun, it often provokes conflict and negative emotions from children, you fear your child's loss of love for you, and it can make you feel rotten. Please try to keep the long-term view in focus. Being a parent sometimes calls for doing things with, to, and for your child that in the short run make the child unhappy but in the long run make him or her better adjusted and happier.

Also remember that all good parents discipline their children. Look around the next time you are at a fast-food restaurant or store full of parents and children. Most parents are correcting their children's misbehavior. Indeed, we often become very judgmental about those who are not doing so.

Besides, the conflicts of this week are quite temporary. Over the next two weeks, time-outs will decrease in frequency and duration as your child learns that the more quickly she becomes quiet the sooner she gets out of the chair. Your child's respect for you—as adults who mean what they say yet are also positive, appreciative, caring, and rewarding—will increase over this time as well.

Finally, understand that the most important role you play as parents from the standpoint of the community is that you, and only you, are the vehicles through which we socialize our children to enter that larger community as good, law-abiding citizens. There is no more important parental role than this once we get past the jobs of feeding, clothing, and nurturing our children. To abdicate this role as socializing agent because you can't bear to discipline your child is a form of gross negligence as a member of the larger social community. We too often forget this charge from our community to us as parents. Yet it is the bedrock of a society and culture.

CHAPTER 9

Step 5: Use Time-Out with Other Misbehavior

Before . . .

"Please, Corey, let's not have a repeat of yesterday, OK?"

Bonnie heaved a sigh as she turned to watch her five-year-old son methodically dribbling milk from a spoon in an intricate pattern all over the breakfast table. Yesterday had been an endless series of trips to and from the time-out chair, punctuated by tantrums and whining from Corey.

"Stop getting milk everywhere, Corey. I'm not going to ask you again!"

Corey obediently put his spoon back in his cereal bowl, then took a long sip of juice into his straw, lifted the end of the straw out of his glass, and spewed juice in a wide orange splatter across the table.

"Corey!" Bonnie yelled. "I said stop making a mess!"

"No you didn't," her son said triumphantly.

"Corey Jamison, if you don't start acting like a five-year-old instead of a two-year-old, you're going to spend the whole day in that chair again!"

"So what?" yelled Corey. "That's what I do all the time anyway!"

After . . .

"Corey, stop making a mess with your milk right now. Five . . . four . . . three. . . ."

Five-year-old Corey looked his mother in the eye, saw that she was watching him unwaveringly, and started using his spoon for its intended purpose: to eat his cereal.

"Thank you, honey. I like it when you do as I ask." Handing him a dishcloth, she added, "Here—wipe up that milk and then finish your breakfast."

Corey started to twirl the dishcloth around in the air.

"Five . . . four. . . ."

"OK, Mom," her son said with a laugh and wiped up the mess.

When he'd finished his cereal and juice, Corey picked up his dishes and brought them to his mother, who was filling the dishwasher.

"Thanks, Corey! It's great that you remembered to clear your place— let's put an extra five chips in your bank."

Corey grinned at Bonnie and ran out of the kitchen to get his token bank.

How did things go last week? If, as I cautioned, the reintroduction of punishment into your defiant child's life made for a rough seven days, it's time for a review. Step 5 is a period for reflection, troubleshooting, and regrouping. If, like Bonnie in the "before" scenario, you're having trouble with time-out and token penalties, you need to discover where you're going wrong so you can make these tools work well for you. If it's been pretty smooth sailing so far, you can start using time-out to help with one or two more behavior problems this week. First, though, bolster your future efforts by taking a little time to confirm what you're doing right. And if you're among the lucky parents who have seen such vast improvement that no significant behavior problems remain, all you need to do is plan to use time-out whenever you need it, regardless of the offense. Again, remind yourself of what's working for you so that you can keep it up as time goes on.

Behavioral Benchmarks of Success

You probably know whether token penalties and time-out are working for you. First and foremost, your child's behavior should be improving overall. Second, your child should be adapting to the use of time-out. You know you're doing well with punishment so far if you're meeting these criteria:

1. Your child is spending less time in the chair for each offense than at the beginning of Step 4. As Chapter 8 explained, some kids will have to sit in the time-out chair for a few hours the first time they are punished this way, but if the method is proving effective they will quickly comply so as to cut down the period during which they are isolated from everything they find desirable.

2. Your child is beginning to accept time-out as punishment, cutting down on tantrums, complaints, and other fussing while in the time-out chair. Also discussed in Chapter 8 was the fact that many children exhibit extreme righteous indignation at the use of any punishment, especially time-out. Defiant children want what they want when they want it, and so being removed from all that they find interesting and enjoyable is an outrage to them. That, of course, means it also strongly discourages them from perpetrating the "crime" that got them into the chair in the first place. If your child is becoming resigned to time-out, it means you have gotten across your conviction to stand firm and your child knows the only way out is to follow your rules. With some kids, you can almost hear the wheels turning in the silence that has replaced their initial tantrums.

3. Your child is doing what you ask in the time-out-targeted area more often. Has your daughter stuck with her homework for longer and longer periods as the week progressed? Is your son interrupting your phone calls less often now? Have you had to tell your child to put away toys only twice today, compared to 10 times a week ago? Getting a response on your first request and, even better, having your child do what you want without being asked at all are signs that you're using punishment effectively and discriminately.

4. Your child is obeying household rules more often. A harmonious home atmosphere depends to a great extent on everyone's following household rules, whether those are "No slamming doors," "No swearing," or "No snacking in the living room." If your child is starting to tow this line because you have posted a list of the rules and begun to enforce them, your home is probably beginning to feel more like a haven than it has in the past.

5. You're feeling more confident in your abilities as a parent. I don't have to tell you how demoralizing it is to have your requests ignored, your commands defied, or your home turned into a war zone. If you're getting results from punishment along with praise—your child's behavior is starting to improve overall—you also should be feeling less helpless and more competent as a parent.

On a Scale of 1 to 10 . . .

Still not sure where you stand? Then fill out the "Defiance in Various Home Situations" questionnaire from Chapter 1 (page 16) again.

Now compare your newly completed form with the answers you saved earlier. Do you see significant improvement? Overall improvement means you're making general progress, and you should keep up the good work. You may also notice certain areas in which improvement has not occurred or is not as great. Those would be the ideal targets for use with time-out this week.

What if you see no improvement to speak of? You've added a brand-new tool to your kit, yet your child's behavior isn't fitting into your home life any better than it used to. Be patient, however. When you are trying to lose weight and have been exercising for only 1 week, you don't get discouraged because you haven't lost 10 pounds yet. So don't get discouraged if your child's behavior is not where you would like it to be. This could take a few more weeks of staying with the program. It's also possible, however, that something is stalling your progress, and you need to find out what it is. Use the following checklist to make sure you are using penalties and time-out as directed:

☐ I am imposing a fine or using time-out *every* time my child is guilty of a particular misbehavior. (Consistency is crucial.)

☐ The fines I impose and the time spent in time-out are in proportion to the severity of the violation. (Fairness is essential.)

☐ The "minimum sentence" that I impose for time-out is based on my child's age. (Realism is necessary.)

☐ My spouse is fining my child in the same way that I am. (Cooperation between parents is important to steady progress.)

☐ I am making sure that my child's fines don't exceed his earnings. (Being "overdrawn" and thus losing all privilege-purchasing power makes the token system useless.)

☐ I stuck to punishing only one or two types of misbehavior during the first week. (Children need time to get used to new forms of discipline if they are to avoid being overwhelmed.)

☐ I've made sure my child can't have any fun while in time-out—no one talks to the child, there are no toys or other forms of entertainment within reach, and the child can't do anything destructive. (If the child's sense of isolation isn't complete, time-out becomes too easy and therefore impotent.)

☐ I never give a command targeted for time-out more than once. (Strict enforcement is the only way to show the child you mean business.)

☐ I am specific in my commands. (If you leave any room for confusion about what you want the child to do, it's unfair to punish him for not doing it.)

☐ I am remembering to count down from five before giving a time-out warning. (Children need this reminder and also a couple of seconds to think through the consequences.)

☐ I am limiting myself to two countdowns from five before giving a time-out. (Waiting too long to impose punishment only gives your anger time to build and encourages overpunishing.)

☐ I never apologize for issuing punishment. (Apologizing sends conflicting messages.)

☐ I always remind my child that I like compliance after the child has given it. (The final thing the child should hear is affirmation of the positive.)

☐ I am remembering to look for behavior to reward soon after imposing punishment. (Always balance punishment with praise.)

A few of you may find that your child's behavior has, after a solid week at Step 4, actually gotten worse—or that the child's behavior remains unchanged, but time-out continues to be a nightmare to enforce. In these cases, your problems may extend beyond the capabilities of self-help, and I strongly suggest that you take this opportunity to get professional help; see Chapter 3.

At my clinic, we spend most of the session devoted to Step 5 on troubleshooting. Many subtle nuances and unimagined glitches can enter into the use of punishment during the first week or so. Because it's difficult to anticipate the solutions you will need, I offer a varied collection of wisdom from the trenches. Now that we are wrapping up the at-home portion of the program, this is also a good time to look at how all the pieces—attention, praise, rewards, penalties, and punishment—are fitting together.

Trouble Spots and Stumbling Blocks

"My son's favorite weapon is to mock me and his father to let us know how little he values our authority. The other day, his reaction to being sent to time-out was to do a headstand in the chair. How can we hope to make any progress this way?"

First of all, I hope you fined him for this behavior during time-out. Unless you take the tack that every action of your child's must have a reaction from you, the entire incentive/disincentive system will fall apart. By doing a headstand, your son was definitely trying to provoke you, and the only thing he should get for his efforts is the negative, consistent consequences you have set this week.

Second, I hope you took the opportunity to have a good laugh over this—in private, that is. I'm sure your son was also trying to be funny, and as long as you don't let your humor deter you from following through, you should take every chance you get to grab the release that laughter brings. If you can show your son that you appreciate his joke while still enforcing the consequences, so much the better.

"My daughter is only four, and it's hard to tell how she is really reacting to time-out. She seems kind of depressed—subdued and sometimes irritable. The other day we caught her giving her teddy bear a time-out for 'being bad,' and her demeanor as the 'parent' was pretty harsh. If that's how she sees us, aren't we doing more harm than good?"

I doubt it. In fact, using this method to discipline her own charges is a strong sign that your daughter feels time-out is effective. Her harshness in acting out your role is probably her way of dealing with any remaining anger over being punished. The key is whether this playacting is accompanied by an improvement in behavior as measured by the five benchmarks listed previously. If it is not, you have some reason for concern and should review your use of the time-out method. Any items in the list on pages 174–175 that you did not check off are areas to target for improvement in your use of time-out. Also, reread Chapter 8 if you have any doubts that you have the process down.

"Last week, when I was about to send my son to time-out, he would immediately promise to do what I had requested. Should I let him comply and avoid the penalty for not listening?"

No! The purpose of your counting backward from five to one after both your request and your subsequent warning is to give the child some time to start to comply. If he has not started by then, he should be sent to time-out, even if along the way he finally decides he should now comply. To do otherwise will teach your child to push you to the very edge of punishment with every command you give just to see if he can get away with it. You want him to respond to your commands or warnings. Although it seems reasonable to let your child comply when he finally relents on his way to time-out, you should follow through by going ahead with the time-out.

"When Antonio was in time-out last week, he repeatedly said that he hated me and didn't love me anymore. I already feel guilty about the fact that Antonio's father left us last year and I had to divorce him; so now Antonio has no father to do things with him. I couldn't bear it if Antonio really did not love me anymore."

Your feelings are quite understandable. But that does not mean that you should avoid fulfilling your responsibility as a parent to discipline Antonio when he needs it. One way, in fact, that children recognize our love and concern for them is that we care enough to punish them when they deserve it. Although they may not appreciate this at the very moment, they do come to understand it later and value your integrity for having cared enough to show them the right and wrong ways to behave. Proper disciplining of a child is like an investment in both your and their future.

Also keep in mind that Antonio may have sensed your insecurities and uncertainties about disciplining him because of your family situation. And he is not above using what he has sensed about you to his own advantage. So you must be sure that your child is not manipulating you out of appropriate discipline by "pushing your emotional buttons" with those phrases he thinks may alarm you and cause you to give in. You can show your love to Ricky later through closer and more positive attention for the good things he surely does with you. But you must also show him your love by following through on your promises to discipline him should he disobey you.

"Shaka went to time-out at least 10 times last week. During some of those times, when I went to ask her if she was ready to do as I asked, she looked at me angrily and just said 'No!' Is this a sign that my use of time-out is failing?"

Absolutely not. There are simply going to be times when your child is so frustrated that she did not get her own way or get out of doing something she really did not want to do that she will take longer to finally give in and agree to comply with you. When your child is in time-out and says no to you–that she is not ready to comply–just say, "Fine, then you sit there until you decide to do as I asked." Eventually your child will consent to do what you asked her to do much earlier in this sequence than she may be doing now. Ultimately, she will just do as you ask and avoid going to time-out altogether. But this training of your child takes some time. Be patient. You'll see that she will come around. Quit now, and you really could be doing harm to your child's future well-being.

"OK. So I did what you said. I caught Andrei hitting his little sister, so I told him to stop it, then counted backward from five. He still hit her again, so I warned him and counted backward from five. Then he stopped. But he still found times to hit her again frequently this past week. Nothing's changed except that I warn him a lot and seem to be counting backward a lot. He stops then, but later he does it again, so I wind up warning him again. What's wrong here?"

It seems you may have misunderstood something we said in the last step. There are two kinds of rules we want children to follow. One type can be considered our instructions and requests. These are things we want a child to do at the time we ask them to do them, like pick up toys. The other type are "household rules." These we don't want to keep repeating. They are rules that are always in effect about how we expect our children to behave. Other household rules might be not to lie, steal, swear, use other people's valued things without permission, take food without asking, and so forth. "No hitting" is a household rule. So, tell your child the next time he hits his little sister he will go to time-out. From that day on, whenever he hits her, he goes immediately to time-out. No commands, no warnings, no backward counting. Zip! Straight to time-out. This should stop the hitting.

"We had to use time-out with Tasha only a few times last week for not picking up her toys when asked. But I'm worried. When she went to the chair for time-out, she seemed very sad and complained aloud that she can't seem to do anything right. She said that she deserved to be punished for everything she does. At one point she even said she hated herself. Is this normal?"

No, it isn't, but just because it's rare does not mean that it's a serious problem. It is possible that Tasha has learned that it bothers you when she talks "depressed" like this and verbally beats herself up for you. Just as Antonio above learned from his mother to say he hated her because it seemed to get him more sympathy and out of time-out sooner, so Tasha may be learning that verbal self-abuse gets your sympathy and that you may be letting her out of time-out sooner as a result. Make sure you are not encouraging your child to make certain verbal statements just to get your sympathy and to avoid punishment.

However, if Tasha seems quite sad more than half of the time for more than two weeks, she could be becoming clinically depressed. If she is saying that she wishes she were dead, you need to take this very seriously. Either way, you need to get professional assistance for her if her sadness extends beyond just being upset in time-out. This is especially true if depression runs in your own or your husband's family.

If it seems that Tasha may be developing depression, stop using the time-out procedure. Concentrate for the time being on your special time, attention to her good behavior, and the use of tokens as rewards

for the good things she does. And get her some professional help as
soon as possible.

*"Jerome was in time-out last week late one afternoon because he would not
start his homework when I asked him to do so. While he was sitting in the
corner, his dad came in from work. His dad went over to him and said, 'Hey,
big guy, what's going on here? Get in your mother's hair, did you? Well,
that's OK. You've had enough time there—let's go throw the baseball around
to get ready for your game tomorrow.' Well, I was furious. But my husband
said that Jerome is his son, too, and that he should be able to overrule my
time-outs if he thinks they have been long enough. Who's right here?"*

You are. It was wrong for your husband to interfere with your disciplining of your son. This can only teach Jerome that Dad's opinion
on punishment matters most and that your threats and discipline
don't count for much. You need to have a talk with your husband outside of Jerome's earshot about this problem. Let him know you understand that he is happy to see Jerome when he comes home and eager
to do things with his son, but all that should wait until Jerome's penalty has been served. Get your husband to understand that you won't
interfere with his disciplining of Jerome when he has to send Jerome to
time-out, and he should not interfere with yours. If this had been a
hockey game and Jerome was in the penalty box for some violation of
the rules, his dad would not go down to that box and tell his son he
could leave it before his penalty was up. He should not do it here, either. That's the referee's call. When you are doing the disciplining, you
are the referee, and it's your call as to when time-out is up. Next time
Jerome is in time-out when your husband comes home, meet him at
the door, smile, and put your finger over your lips to immediately signal to him that he needs to come in quietly while Jerome serves his
time-out.

*"My nine-year-old son will impulsively get out of the time-out chair because
he is upset. What should I do?"*

Here is an intriguing strategy devised by one father: He and his
son made a "For Sale" sign with the letters actually cut out of ply-
wood with a jigsaw. The sign was kept with the boy's beloved dirt
bike. Each time the boy got out of the time-out chair, he lost a letter. If

he successfully stayed in the chair for the entire time-out, he earned a letter back. If he lost all the letters from the sign, the dirt bike would be sold.

"My child refuses to apologize for hitting his brother after time-out is over. What should I do?"

For some children, the act of verbally apologizing to a sibling is perceived as not only stressful but humiliating. One family I know decided instead to have the child write a short note to his brother as a condition for time-out to be terminated.

"My eight-year-old daughter refuses to sit in the time-out chair, despite being fined a large number of chips. What recourse do I have left?"

When a child refuses to stay in the chair, you have three options. If the child is physically very small, you can kneel down behind the chair and wrap your arms around the child, actually holding her physically in the chair—an approach typically used with four- or five-year-olds. For older children (especially 11- or 12-year-olds), "grounding"—in which the child loses access to anything you would define as a privilege for a brief period of time (three or four hours up to 1 full day)—is more appropriate. For children in between these ages, such as your eight-year-old, inform the child that if she refuses to stay in the time-out chair, her room will be stripped of all toys, games, books, and so forth so that time-out can be served in the child's room.

"My child is 11 years old and seems too mature to sit in a time-out chair."

In the case of older children who may seem too mature or sophisticated to sit in an isolated chair, having the child sit at the dining room table or on the stairs from the first to the second floor of the house is perfectly acceptable. As long as the child is out of the mainstream of household activity and is not being entertained while sitting out, the time-out purpose is served.

"My child is constantly calling to me and asking me questions while he is in time-out, and he gets even more upset when I don't respond to him. What should I do?"

Time-out means "time out from reinforcement." Having a dialogue with a parent can be quite rewarding (reinforcing) for many children. Therefore, you should not be discussing or debating with your child during time-out. Explain to your child ahead of time that you will not be talking to him while he is in time-out and make sure the child understands this. If the child seems to become more upset while in time-out and calls out to you, ignore it as long as the child does not leave the chair.

"My child complains bitterly that time-out is unfair because grown-ups don't have to do it."

Rather than getting into a long, philosophical discussion about the status of children and adults, one family allowed their son to write a "contract" for them where they as parents agreed that they would be as fair as possible in using time-out. The son stipulated that he would reward them for their fairness with a "prize" at the end of six months. This process allowed the boy to save face, and he accepted time-out much more willingly.

CHAPTER 10

Step 6: Think Aloud and Think Ahead— What to Do in Public

Before . . .

"Brendan, wait," Malika pleaded as her seven-year-old son tumbled out of the car. "I don't want a repeat of yesterday, young man, so please try to be-have."

"OK, Mom," Brendan said, and then he shot off across the parking lot, reaching the hardware store 20 yards ahead of his mother.

As Malika caught up with him, she grabbed his wrist and yanked him back toward her. "Remember, be good," she said.

Her son flashed her a big grin and ran inside the store, where he immediately began zigzagging down one of the aisles, picking up this and grabbing that, occasionally knocking an item off a shelf.

"Brendan," his mother hissed. "Come back here this minute." Anxiously Malika looked around to see who was watching them. "If I have to pay for anything you break today, there won't be any TV for a whole week!"

"OK, Mom," Brendan said in disgust as he grabbed a pole, spun around . . . and around . . . and around . . . until his momentum was halted when he slammed into an unsuspecting shopper.

"I'm so sorry," Malika said, cringing. Turning to her son, she said un-der her breath, "Do not embarrass me again, Brendan."

"Mom," Brendan whined, "it was an accident. It wasn't my fault!" As he stamped his feet, his arms flailed out toward the sacks of weed killer stacked at the intersection of two aisles, knocking off the top three bags and spewing the contents of one of them all over the floor.

Trying to avoid the patronizing gaze of the clerk who started sweeping up the mess, Malika cringed, gritted her teeth, and dragged her son out of the store without the brackets and screws she'd intended to buy.

"Just wait till I get you home," she seethed, all eyes on them as they skulked out.

After . . .

"Brendan, stop!" Malika yelled when she saw her son start to pull the hardware store door open. Catching up to him, she pulled him to the side and said, "Now remember what we discussed at home, Brendan: When we go in, you stay with me, don't touch anything, and be quiet. If you can do that the whole time we're inside, you'll get 10 chips. If you don't do that, you'll lose 10. Can you tell me what the rules are?"

"Sure," Brendan said. "Stay with you, no touching, no yelling."

"You can help me, too, if you can find the hardware for the shelves we're putting up. I bet you'll spot the bins with the screws in them before I do. You've got great eyes. OK?"

"OK, Mom," Brendan said as he took his mother's hand and led her inside the store.

Brendan did just fine for about two minutes, then, in his eagerness to help find the screws his mother needed, he pulled away and started to run down the aisle.

"Brendan!" his mother called. "Stop right now or you'll lose 10 chips!"

"But Mom . . . " Brendan protested as he rounded the corner and slipped out of sight.

When Malika spotted him, she said, "OK, Brendan, you've lost the chips. Come back here and follow the rules."

"That's not fair!" her son shouted, and threw a handful of screws on the floor.

Malika walked up to her son, took him firmly by the arm, and escorted him to a nearby corner of the store where none of the store's goods were within reach. Turning her son to face the unadorned wall, she instructed, "Stand *there quietly until I say you can move." She then set her watch for three minutes as she looked over the screws to find the size she needed.*

When the time was up, she retrieved her son and quietly told him to help her pick up the screws he had thrown.

Her son quickly cleaned up the mess, took his mother's hand, and offered to carry her bag after they had paid for their purchases.

Malika and Jesse Harrison had thought they had it made. The combination of rewards and mild, consistent punishment had transformed their home from a battle zone to the haven it always should have been. Why, then, did Brendan revert to the terror he used to be whenever they left the house?

Because even parents who use the home token system and timeout with great success often have a hard time taking what they've learned with them into the wider world. Maybe, like Malika before she went through Step 6, you're a paragon of fairness, attentiveness, and consistency at home. But something happens when you go out in public. With all the uncontrollable factors operating out there, you know anything can happen, and this makes you lose a little of your confidence. Besides, out there beyond the confines of your own home, *people are watching.*

"Wait till I get you home" resonates for most of us. Our own parents taught us not to "air our dirty laundry" in public, and many of our old methods of managing our children certainly fell into the category of dirty laundry. It *is* embarrassing to be stared at while threatening, berating, or spanking your child in public. Fortunately, you no longer need to resort to such coercion to control your child. You're already applying more effective methods at home, and in this chapter you'll learn how to make them work for you when you're away, whether shopping, worshiping, dining, or visiting. I also tell you how to use these methods to make those trying special occasions at home, like holiday events, manageable as well.

Getting over any anticipated embarrassment is a big hurdle for some parents, but a little experience will demonstrate that exercising reasonable control over your child in public is nothing to be ashamed of. You might , in fact, find yourself getting admiring glances rather than critical looks. It's only what you deserve when you show that you can manage your child's misbehavior quickly and with minimal intrusion on those around you.

Having tried the alternative, you know that waiting to impose consequences never works for children like yours. But, many parents protest, if I don't wait till we get home I'm likely to overreact, because my child's misbehavior always takes me by surprise. My response is: Don't let yourself be taken entirely by surprise. Anticipating problems is a great antidote to the flustered, humiliated feeling that overtakes us when our Dr. Jekyll at home turns into Mr. Hyde in public.

Thinking ahead can go a long way toward keeping the unpredictable from becoming unmanageable. Thinking aloud can go a long way toward reminding your child that you expect the same good behavior you expect at home even when the setting has changed. As Malika in the "after" scenario illustrated, the inevitable little transgressions don't have to mushroom into disasters if you tell your child what to expect immediately before entering a public place. Many parents find reminding their child that both good and bad behavior away from home will have consequences deters the child from behaving poorly in public. That depends, however, on the child's faith that you will enforce the rules you set. When your child knows you mean what you say at home, it doesn't take long for him to figure out that you'll be just as dependable in other places. In fact, many parents find that after Step 5 all they need to do to discourage defiant behavior in public is to state the rules and the penalties beforehand and then intermittently hand out praise (and chips or points) for good behavior as they go along. They never even need time-out as Malika did in the "after" scenario.

Here's an overview of how Step 6 can get you to that point:

*1. **Think ahead.*** Anticipate places and times when your child is likely to have trouble behaving—and also where you might be prone to losing your aplomb. Come up with realistic expectations for your child's behavior in these situations: rules to be followed, consequences for following or violating them, and activities to keep your child diverted while you're out.

*2. **Think aloud.*** Stop before entering any public place and communicate these rules, consequences, and activities to your child.

3. Impose the consequences while away from home, remembering to offer praise and incentives often and imposing reasonable punishment without embarrassment when needed.

4. Start applying the same techniques to major transitions in the child's activities or special events at home.

First, the preliminaries:

Where Are You Likely to Have Trouble with Your Child?

Take a few minutes to sit down with a sheet of paper and jot a list of places, times, or situations where your child is likely to act in a defiant or other problematic manner. Parents usually know where their children are most likely to break the rules of behavior. Is your child driven wild by the candy section of the supermarket? Does your child find it impossible to resist playing with every item at the local toy store? Can your daughter sit still and be quiet at your place of worship? Can your son dine out in a somewhat civilized manner? I'm sure you have a long mental record of past incidents that will tell you where to expect problems.

Are excursions easier at certain times of day than at others? Maybe your daughter is perfectly fine grocery shopping early Saturday morning but a whirling dervish if expected to contain herself at any store after sitting at her desk in school all day. Kids who still take naps will probably not be at their best if you time an errand to occur right before (or during!) their usual naptime. A child may balk at a 45-minute car ride unless some active playtime is scheduled first.

Other elements need to be considered, too. Does your child do better with a friend or sibling along for company, or does companionship just provide the child with a likely "partner in crime"? If your child tends to be irritable or touchy, the same place may affect her differently under varying circumstances: Will a crowded movie theater pose a greater challenge than an empty one? Your astute understanding of what bothers and soothes your child can help you accurately foresee potential problems.

When Do Your Most Embarrassing Moments Occur?

Fear of embarrassment can definitely stand in the way of managing your child's behavior in public places, so you need to anticipate your own reactions to potential problems. Take out another sheet of paper and write down the types of places where you're most likely to be embarrassed by any "scenes" caused by your child. Some parents won't bat an eye at misbehavior in the grocery store but are mortified by any peep out of their child at church. Others don't mind noise or overactivity in public but can't tolerate rudeness. What pushes your buttons? Whatever causes you anxiety and embarrassment also threatens your ability to stay cool in managing your child. These situations call for extra precautions—possibly extra incentives and diversions to encourage good behavior and an extra repetition of the rules before entering the public place. And if they really make you nervous, you may not want to use these situations as test cases as suggested later in this chapter—at least not until you've gained a little confidence in other settings.

Rest assured, however, that the success you have already achieved at home has a way of automatically transferring to other venues. Credibility is a powerful asset. Knowing that you will indeed impose the defined consequences for misbehavior usually discourages your child from acting out in the first place. And if something does go awry, as long as you're willing to take swift, decisive action, the disruption should be much less than it has been in the past. The best way to confirm this is to try it, so let's get started.

What to Do in Public

1. State the rules to your child immediately before entering a public place. The first time out, stop directly before going into the store, temple, restaurant, or other public place and tell your child the rules. Keep it simple and succinct, such as "Stand close, don't touch, and don't beg!" for a store. For a place of worship it might be "Hands to yourself and don't talk!" For older children the rules can be a little more complicated—"Stay in your seat, don't touch your sister, and use your silverware" for a restaurant—but don't forget the principle of specifici-ty that you learned way back in Chapter 4. Malika in the "before" sce-nario at the beginning of this chapter made the mistake of using gener-alities like "Don't embarrass me" and "Be good," as well as making vague references to what had happened yesterday. When you're out in public, it's crucial not to leave the rules up to the child's interpretation.

Now have your child repeat the rules back to you to be sure he or she heard and understood.

If you thought ahead as advised, you had an idea of what the rules should be for regularly visited venues like grocery stores. You can adapt them to fit individual circumstances, but try to establish cer-tain rules that you will always want your child to follow in the store. Then, the next time you go to the store, you need only ask outside, "What are the rules?" If your child can't remember, restate them and ask the child to repeat them.

2. Offer an incentive for cooperation. The easiest incentive to of-fer your child for obeying the rules you've just stated is a certain num-ber of chips or points from the token system. They can either be dis-pensed periodically during the outing or all at once at the end, but if the latter, be sure to praise your child often for obeying the rules dur-ing the trip. If your child is so young that you're not using the home token system, you can take along a little bag of treats and tell the child outside the store that you'll be dispensing the treats for cooperation while in the public place. If either of these ideas is impractical, or when you need an added incentive on top of these, you can promise the child some other reward at the end of the trip ("If you follow the rules in the store, you'll get 10 points, and, because I know it's so easy to get excited in a toy store so close to Hanukkah, we'll stop and rent a video on the way home"). Please use this incentive selectively, though, or your child may expect you to spend money on him after every trip during which he cooperates!

3. Explain what the punishment will be for failing to cooperate. Again, the simplest approach is to deduct tokens—"You'll lose 10 points if you disobey the rules while we're eating dinner"—but you should also be prepared to use time-out. This is where many parents hesitate, believing that time-out is either impractical or inappropriate in public. I assure you that it's not impractical, because the places you frequent are undoubtedly familiar enough to you that you can identify a dull corner easily. Nor is time-out inappropriate. No one wants to appear "cruel" to onlooking strangers, but having your child stand quietly in a boring spot is much less cruel than dragging him away or screaming at him. Again, most onlookers will appreciate your efforts to prevent your child from imposing on them in public.

Tips for using time-out effectively in public follow these instructions. Whatever consequence you tell your child will follow misbehavior, make sure it's specific, sensible, and defined ahead of time. In the "before" scenario, Brendan did not believe his mother would carry out her threat to take away his TV privileges for a week because the punishment was out of proportion to the "crime" and obviously flowed from the heat of the moment rather than rational thought. Once you do have to impose a consequence, do it immediately, without repeating commands or rules or negotiating with the child. As at home, negotiating and offering "one more chance" will only rob you of credibility in imposing future consequences.

4. Give your child something to do. All kids love to help their parents, and they all appreciate being given a useful task that will also stave off boredom during a trip or errand that is your idea rather than theirs. This should be a particularly fun part of your outings for both you and your child. If the child is old enough, take some time on the way to the store to ask her for ideas of how she can help. Also have some ideas of your own—helping you find something on the shelves, checking things off on your grocery list, carrying a small bag, or unloading your cart are just a few possibilities for a store. At a restaurant, consider asking your defiant child to help entertain a younger sibling by playing "I spy with my little eye" while waiting for your food to be brought to the table. Or, at church, ask your child to turn the pages of the hymnal for you. Use your imagination. Unstructured situations beg to be filled, and you won't always approve of how your child chooses to plug the gap. Activities planned by parents, on the other hand, have been proven to reduce disruptive behavior.

Start this week by making two trial runs out into the great wide world. Choose two typically problematic public places—maybe one from your list of problematic situations for your child and one from your list of situations in which you're most uncomfortable with discipline—and stage a trip there for the sole purpose of using the method just described. These rehearsals should prove to you how effective the techniques can be. And if you run into any hitches, nothing will be lost: You won't have frustrated your attempts to shop for dinner or missed a sorely needed meal out. Once you've had a relatively successful run-through, you can start using these measures in "real life."

Using Time-Out When You're Out

1. The first thing you should do when you enter a public place is scan the area for a potential time-out spot if you don't already know of one. Likely spots are listed in the box on page 192. If there is no viable place for time-out, try one of these alternatives:

- Quickly take the child outside and impose the time-out against a wall.
- Take the child back to the car, where the child sits in the back seat or on the floor of the back seat while you stay in the front seat or right outside the car.
- Carry a notebook for recording rule violations, and explain to the child, along with the rules, that for every violation recorded the child will serve a minimum sentence in time-out at home.
- Carry a marker or pen and put a light hash mark on the child's hand for every violation. Each mark counts as a minimum sentence in time-out at home.

2. When the child violates a rule, immediately take him to the designated spot and tell the child to stay there until you say he can leave. Follow the same procedure as at home, except that the child needs to stay in this spot for only 30 seconds for every year of age. Shorter time-outs usually are just as great a deterrent in public since there are many more attractive diversions around the child—and because many children are as embarrassed by being in time-out as their parents expect to be! While the child is in time-out, stay close enough to supervise but occupy yourself with some activity, such as checking over your grocery list, looking at items on the shelves, and so on.

3. When the child has served the sentence, been quiet for a minute, and agreed to comply with the broken rule from now on, you can "spring" her. But if she "escapes" before the time is up, start over and tell her that she will lose a certain number of points if she does it again. If she does escape again, fine her the points as stated and keep returning her to time-out until she cooperates. If you find you're getting nowhere, you may have to interrupt your trip and take the child out to the car to serve the time-out, supervised by you.

Punishment during Long Car Trips

A long car trip with a defiant, possibly overactive, child can be a nightmare of spats with siblings, tests to find out if you can drive and discipline at the same time, and endless repetitions of "Are we there yet?" It doesn't have to be that bad if you use the Step 6 methods. As described earlier, review the rules before setting out, take along plenty of diversions (games or toys, plus ideas for fun activities like spotting out-of-state license plates or unusual car models or singing songs), and state the consequences for breaking the rules. Points or chips can

---

GOOD SPOTS FOR TIME-OUT IN PUBLIC

In a department store: Facing the dull side of a display counter or a corner of a relatively vacant aisle; facing a rack of coats; a dull corner in a customer service or other nonsales department; a dull corner of a rest room; a nearby fitting room; a maternity section—where you'll find fewer customers, all of whom will probably be sympathetic mothers!

In a grocery store: Facing the frozen food counter; in the most remote corner of the store; facing the dull side of a counter in the greeting card section while you look at the cards.

In a place of worship: In the vestibule, rest room, or "crying room" designated for fussy babies.

In a restaurant: Rest rooms are usually the only practical choice.

In other people's homes: In any chair or corner designated by a cooperative host, whom you have told about your new child management method upon arriving.

be deducted as they are anywhere else. *Do not try to implement time-out while driving.* Some parents believe they have their child captive and so time-out should be easy, but you can't possibly supervise adequately and drive safely. If you need to impose time-out, pull over to a safe spot like a shopping mall parking lot and have the child serve the time-out in the back seat or on a floor mat outside the car. *Never leave the child unattended, whether in the car or outside.*

Thinking Ahead and Thinking Aloud in Other Situations

Defiant children often have difficulty making the transitions required of them, whether it's from playtime to bedtime, from a quiet home to one teeming with relatives, or from doing anything they like to doing anything they don't like. Take out a third sheet of paper and jot down all the big transitions that your child typically has trouble with. Include not only transitions to disliked activities—playtime to homework time, TV time to bath time, outdoor time to dinner time—but also those to activities the child anticipates with great pleasure. A defiant child who is excited about having a friend over, having a birthday party, or having grandparents or cousins arrive for a holiday is always at risk for boiling over or falling apart. Calm things down by gently but firmly telling the child what you expect in the form of rules and the consequences for upholding or breaking them. Be sensitive to your child's efforts to keep it together in trying circumstances like holiday mania and offer extra praise or even extra rewards.

Trouble Spots and Stumbling Blocks

"It's just not worth it for me to try to come up with a real job my son can do to help me when we're out. He always seems to make a mess of it, no matter how hard he tries, and I just end up madder at him than I would be if he just broke the rules. What should I do?"

Although it really is great for a kid's self-esteem to be of help, kids can spot a setup a mile away. Your son probably knows you're doing him a favor rather than entrusting him with a responsibility when you ask him to help in these situations, and "making a mess of it" may even be his defiant way of showing you how he feels about your lack of candor. Forget about coming up with a job for him and just focus on finding something diverting for him to do. Experience has shown that any assigned activity is better than nothing, even if it isn't particularly constructive. Go all out with your imagination. Instead of asking him to find the peanut butter brand that you like at the grocery store, tell him that Martians are coming to earth to collect all the food that little kids don't like, and he can help them take it away by pointing out each food on the shelves that he'd like to see disappear from the planet.

"I hate to set up extra rules for my son at Christmas. He's so excited and so happy, and I'm afraid being tougher on him with all the company in the house will be a disaster. Any tips?"

Actually, many families suspend some of their regular rules and lighten up on the consequences during special events like holidays. In one of the parent groups we ran around Thanksgiving, several couples decided that the commotion of a large family gathering called for a modified public-places approach to discipline. They would choose only two or three important rules (such as "no running in the house"), which would be conveyed on Thanksgiving morning, right before the relatives arrived. Tokens would be earned or lost only for those few rules and not for the usual household rules. Any time-out served would also be shortened to the 30-seconds-per-year-of-age duration. This is a great example of thinking ahead, forming realistic expectations, and adapting to the situation at hand.

"We've virtually stopped taking driving vacations because of all the bickering that goes on in the back seat, but this year we have to go to a family reunion that's hundreds of miles away. What type of incentive do you recommend for a kid who just can't behave in the car?"

I'll pass on an ingenious bit of wisdom from one family who had a similar problem: On their long car trip to visit grandparents, they told their son he could earn 25 cents for every 15 minutes that passed without his arguing with anyone, and he could spend the money during their visit. The $20 that his parents had to shell out at their destination was, they swore, the best money they had ever spent.

"When we go on a trip, we're traveling with a full car. Where is everyone else supposed to go when our son needs to serve a time-out in the car?"

One family thought ahead on this one: The parents bought a stack of magazines—rock music and fashion magazines for their teenager, comic books for their middle child, and news magazines for the adults—which they stashed out of sight until a time-out was called for. Then, when they stopped at a rest stop, they pulled out the magazines as a surprise and read them in the front and back seats while their little boy sat in the cargo area of their sports utility vehicle with nothing to do. Four minutes of this was plenty to keep his behavior under control for the next couple of hours.

"My child has been getting away with murder in public for years. What makes you think she'll take my discipline seriously now?"

She won't if you still waffle at home, but if you've been sticking to your guns in the house, your child should now be convinced that you mean what you say. You may be surprised by how little your daughter will challenge your authority in public now that you've fully demonstrated your willingness to impose time-out as you say you will.

"Since time-out and fines have worked so well for us at home, why can't we just make it clear to our child that any misbehavior in public will mean punishment when we get back home?"

For most children, this "wait until I get you home" approach just isn't compelling. They need immediate, quick action from you in response to misbehavior—just as they need quick affirmation of good behavior. Many defiant children, especially if they have ADHD, can't retain the thought of what will happen later in a fashion that will govern their behavior now. That's why you've been using tokens and time-out at home: to hammer home the idea that every action has a consistent, predictable reaction from you—positive or negative. If, for whatever reason, you simply cannot impose consequences on the spot, recording violations in a notebook or using hash marks on the child's hand serves as an immediate response holding the promise of a significant consequence later.

"I just can't interrupt our church services to impose time-out. I even feel funny talking about point penalties when I should be listening to the sermon, but my daughter just ignores me when I try to put hash marks on her hand. What else can I do?"

Some kind of more immediate reminder of what's in store at home may sink in and prove a more powerful deterrent. Some kids find the reminder of seeing marks on the back of their hand visually reinforcing enough. Others don't. For them, I have found that showing them a photo of themselves sitting in the time-out chair brings it all into focus. To make this tool effective, be sure you show it to your daughter before entering church, when you tell her that every hash mark she gets means a time-out the minute you get home.

CHAPTER 11

Step 7: Help the Teacher Help Your Child

Before . . .

". . . Thanks, Ms. Santos. I'll talk to my husband about this and get back to you right away. Believe me, we do take this problem seriously. I'm glad you called."

"Jack, get down here this minute!" Janet yelled after hanging up the kitchen phone. Her nine-year-old son came thundering down the stairs and then stood stock-still when he saw the look on his mother's face.

"What?" Jack asked cautiously.

"I just heard from your teacher, Jack. I understand you had a little trouble on the playground today?"

Jack gulped and nodded.

"And then you disrupted the entire class during the science quiz, forcing Ms. Santos to give the test over tomorrow?"

"It wasn't my fault, Mom," Jack whined, shuffling his feet and beginning to bang his hand against the kitchen door frame. "I got finished early and I just couldn't stand it—I was so bored!"

"Jack, that's no excuse for making noise, throwing spitballs, and keeping the other kids from concentrating when they need to. And that test you 'finished'—Ms. Santos said you got a 60 on it! You've been so great around here—what's happened to you?"

"I don't know, Mom," Jack said, hanging his head.

"Well, I'll have to talk to Dad about this, but I can tell you one thing: All privileges are off for today."

"Mom," Jack protested.

"No arguments!" his mother snapped as she turned back to the wall phone and started dialing.

"Oh, hi, honey," Janet said as her son trudged back up the stairs. "Well, I guess the honeymoon is over. . . ."

After . . .

"It's four o'clock, Jack," Janet said as she peered around the corner into the kitchen. "Finish up your snack and come into the dining room so we can go over your report for today."

Jack pulled a sheet of paper from his backpack and joined his mother. Heaving a big sigh as he handed her the paper, he said, "I didn't do so great today, Mom."

"Oh?" his mother answered mildly. "Let's take a look."

After perusing the paper briefly, she looked up at her son and said, "I see you got two 1's today, honey. That's terrific! Fifty points is a lot to add to your checkbook."

Taking a moment to compose herself before going on, Janet glanced back down at the paper and then said, "You had some trouble on the playground today, I see. Tell me what happened."

"It was that Patrick Custer's fault, Mom, honest! He kept pushing and pushing when Mr. Jonas wasn't looking, and I finally let him have it!"

"You know hitting is strictly against the rules—here and at school—Jack. And I'm sure right now it doesn't seem worth the 25 points it cost you."

"That Patrick oughtta be the one to lose the points," Jack muttered angrily. Janet ignored him and kept her voice calm: "I guess things went downhill after recess, Jack. Ms. Santos is pretty upset about having to regive the science quiz tomorrow because of your behavior. What happened there?"

"That test was easy," Jack answered. "I got finished before everyone else and I got really bored. I couldn't just sit there forever like that!"

"Jack, that behavior got you another 5 from Ms. Santos, which means you lose another 25 points. And, by the way, Ms. Santos took the trouble to grade your quiz before you went home, and she's written here on the back that you got a 60 on it, so obviously you weren't as 'finished' as you thought."

"What?!" Jack cried indignantly.

"Sit down, Jack. Let's see how you can handle both situations differently tomorrow. It's a shame to have those 1's get washed out by 5's, isn't it?"

If you're not getting calls or notes from your child's teacher, and your son or daughter's academic performance is acceptable, you may not need Step 7 right now. Some kids never take their defiant behavior to school with them, and some reap such drastic improvement from Steps 1–6 that their great new behavior flows naturally into the classroom and onto the playground. Please read this chapter anyway, so you're not caught off guard if school problems develop in the future.

How likely your child is to have problems in all settings depends largely on how severe his or her defiant behavior has been. An extremely oppositional child probably argues with his teachers as much as with you or the lifeguard at the community pool; a very defiant child probably breaks school rules along with home and social rules. For those whose behavior falls closer to the middle of the continuum, the likelihood of defiance at school depends on many factors, from how well the school's level of structure fits your child's temperament to the types of social challenges the school poses to the relationship between the child and the teacher(s).

The school day may be smooth sailing for your child right now, but will it remain that way if a new teacher enters the picture, your child moves from elementary school to middle school, or some kind of social strife erupts? Remember, above all, that your defiant child has trouble controlling himself, adapting, and staying calm even in situations that involve only ordinary everyday levels of conflict. As your child grows, and her schools throw new challenges at her, she may very well react with negative behavior.

If your child has been having trouble at school, I'm sure you've already heard about it, and you can put Step 7 to work right away. If not, be prepared to use Step 7 if the need arises and keep in mind that a "relapse" in behavior that shows up at school need not mean the honeymoon is over. It could be just a blip, one that is easily erased by using the plan laid out in this chapter. Most of the parents who consult us are able to phase out their use of this method in a matter of a month or two.

Here's what you will do, now or in the future:

1. When poor behavior at school comes to your attention, discuss with the teacher the "daily school behavior report card" explained in the following pages. Together, the two of you can come to agreement on the specific problems that need to be resolved and exactly how the teacher will report on your child's behavior every day.

2. Explain the system to your child: To help him or her overcome behavior problems that are showing up at school, the teacher will keep track of the child's behavior—in class, on the playground, or both—by sending home a behavior report card every day. You will then review the card, adding or subtracting chips or points from the home token system already in place, according to the "grades" the teacher has given the child for that day.

3. Plan to meet with the teacher every few weeks to discuss progress and review the reports.

4. Plan to put the system into effect for at least a couple of weeks, and then, if it is successful, switch from daily reports to two reports a week and then to one a week or one a month, depending on how effective this step has been, before phasing it out completely.

Gaining the Teacher's Cooperation

To put this plan into effect, you need to get the teacher's cooperation, a task that may require some tact. Before you broach the subject of daily behavior report cards, think about the relationship that you and your child have forged with this teacher so far. Has there been a sense of collaboration (even conspiracy) to help your child? Does the teacher view you as a cooperative parent who is realistic about the child's behavior and sympathetic toward the teacher's job? Has communication between you been constructive? Is the teacher still open to helping your child or exasperated by your child's unrelenting disruptiveness? All of these factors may influence the reception you get when you introduce this plan.

Remember, too, that all teachers have numerous demands on their time and energy, and what you're asking adds yet another one to their list—at least at first. You'll need to convey that *you* will do most of the work, *you* will take responsibility for imposing consequences, and, most important of all, *the teacher* will reap the benefit. Most teachers will jump at an offer like that, especially if they've already tried everything they know to correct your child's school behavior. In fact, you might introduce your plan as a way to enhance the effectiveness of any in-class behavior modification technique the teacher has implemented with disappointing results. We have found that the behavior report card system is as effective as these classroom behavior management techniques, sometimes more effective, and it always makes the in-class methods more effective.

Teachers may try a number of methods to help a defiant child stick with the program, many of which were developed initially for ADHD. Your child's teacher might take simple measures, from seating your child close to the teacher's desk, to posting signs covering rules and putting cards on the child's desk that list the rules for desk work, to having your child restate the rules before a new period or activity begins. We train teachers to use methods very similar to those in this parent program, including paying positive attention and giving effective commands, as well as setting up some sort of token system at school. But often these methods get a major boost when they are supported by the home token system as described in this chapter.

One school awarded children points for appropriate behavior, which could then be redeemed at the school store for pencils, erasers, and other such supplies. The problem with the program, said the parents of a 12-year-old boy at this school, was that he didn't want pencils or anything else available at the store. All he really cared about, they said, was being able to go out in the woods with his friends after school and ride four-wheelers, sneak cigarettes, and look at "girly magazines." Obviously this school behavior modification program did not motivate the boy to improve his behavior. Tying it in with the rewards he was working for at home, however, did.

If you're getting regular calls or notes about your child's behavior, you'll have many natural opportunities to bring up your plan with the teacher. Otherwise, call the teacher and ask for an appointment to come in and talk about what you can do to help the teacher with your child's behavior at school. Tell the teacher that what you have in mind is one step in a program that you've found very helpful in improving your child's behavior at home and in public. Give him or her an overview of the home token system and the principles you've adopted in managing your child if you haven't been discussing the program with the teacher all along.

If the teacher is amenable to the idea, ask if he or she would be willing to fill out the behavior rating forms on pages 205 and 207, as well as the following form, before meeting with you, so you'll both be prepared to zero in on your child's specific problem areas.

BEHAVIOR IN VARIOUS SCHOOL SITUATIONS

To the teacher: Does this child present any problems in complying with instructions, commands, or rules for you in any of these situations? If so, please circle *Yes*, and then circle the number that describes the problem's severity. If not, circle *No*. Then add up the number of problem settings and calculate the average severity score.

Situations	Yes/No		Mild								Severe
When arriving at school	Yes	No	1	2	3	4	5	6	7	8	9
During individual desk	Yes	No	1	2	3	4	5	6	7	8	9
During small group activities	Yes	No	1	2	3	4	5	6	7	8	9
During free playtime in class	Yes	No	1	2	3	4	5	6	7	8	9
During lectures to the class	Yes	No	1	2	3	4	5	6	7	8	9
At recess	Yes	No	1	2	3	4	5	6	7	8	9
At lunch	Yes	No	1	2	3	4	5	6	7	8	9
In the halls	Yes	No	1	2	3	4	5	6	7	8	9
In the bathroom	Yes	No	1	2	3	4	5	6	7	8	9
On field trips	Yes	No	1	2	3	4	5	6	7	8	9
During special assemblies	Yes	No	1	2	3	4	5	6	7	8	9
On the bus	Yes	No	1	2	3	4	5	6	7	8	9

Total number of problem settings _____ Mean severity score _____

When you meet, offer an acknowledgment of your child's behavior problem and your appreciation for the teacher's efforts on the child's behalf. Stress how confident you are that the strides you've made outside of school can be brought into school. Then explain how the report cards work: You will impose consequences at home for your child's behavior at school. All the teacher needs to do is fill out the school behavior report card every day, at least at first. You will see that the child delivers the report card to you and will impose penalties if the child doesn't do so. You will offer incentives for good school behavior by awarding chips or points, and you will offer disincentives for bad behavior by subtracting chips or points.

Now ask the teacher where she (let's assume the teacher is Ms. Santos) sees the greatest behavior problems—during class or during free time, such as recess? Use the forms she has filled out to zero in on more specific problem areas. Show the teacher the report card forms in this chapter—one for class behavior, one for free-time behavior, and one blank form. Discuss which one would be most useful with your child, pointing out that you would like to limit the targeted behaviors to four or five at first, with others to be added as you both agree, once your child is doing well with these initial behaviors. Also explain that you would like to include one or two in which your child stands a pretty good chance of success. This way, as with your home system, the child will not end up so severely penalized for problem behavior that he loses all his points for the day; rather he can take hope from offsetting some of his "failures" with successes.

Ask the teacher whether she would prefer to have you supply a stack of the cards for her use or send one in each day with your child.

Now explain how the report card is to be used: After each class or period, the teacher enters a rating from 1 (for "excellent") to 5 (for "very poor") for each behavior on the card, adding to the back of the card any comments about the behavior, the situation, or the rating assigned. Then the teacher initials the ratings. At the end of the day, the card is to be given to your child to take home and deliver to you.

You and the teacher should discuss whether the ratings should be given for every period of the school day or for only selected class times at first. Some children will benefit from starting small and seeing their achievements in one or two subjects or time periods at first; then the teacher can gradually extend the system to the whole day.

Ask the teacher to be sure to note on the back of the card, or on some separate record if she prefers, any improvements she begins to see in your child's behavior as time goes on. Improvements should be reflected in an increasing number of 1's and 2's on the report cards, of course, but taking the trouble to note improvements in words has a way of cementing your child's progress in the teacher's mind and eliciting that all-important praise from the teacher as well as from you. Tell the teacher that you plan to keep the cards, and ask if you can schedule a meeting with her every couple of weeks or so to review the cards and your child's progress.

POSSIBLE BEHAVIORS TO GRADE

As with the home token system, success with the daily behavior report cards depends on a judicious selection of behaviors to be rated. In addition to the items listed on the forms, the following are behaviors that many parents target. Consider these when working with the teacher to devise your child's report card.

Social conduct

- Shares with classmates
- Plays well with peers
- Follows rules during playtime
- Cooperates in groups
- Stays in assigned seat
- Works/plays quietly
- Arrives on time for classes
- Maintains an orderly desk and locker

Academic performance

- Completes math [reading, science, social studies, etc.] assignments
- Takes homework assignments home
- Completes homework
- Brings completed homework back to school on time

(cont. on p. 208)

DAILY SCHOOL BEHAVIOR REPORT CARD

Child's name_____ Date_____

Teachers:
Please rate this child's behavior today in the areas listed below. Use a separate column for each subject or class period. Use the following ratings: 1 = excellent, 2 = good, 3 = fair, 4 = poor, and 5 = very poor. Then initial the box at the bottom of your column. Add any comments about the child's behavior today on the back of this card.

Behaviors to be rated:	Class periods/subjects						
	1	2	3	4	5	6	7
Class participation							
Performance of class work							
Follows classroom rules							
Gets along well with other children							
Quality of homework, if any given							
Teacher's initials							

Place comments on back of card

- Cut here after photocopying -

DAILY SCHOOL BEHAVIOR REPORT CARD

Child's name_____ Date_____

Teachers:
Please rate this child's behavior today in the areas listed below. Use a separate column for each subject or class period. Use the following ratings: 1 = excellent, 2 = good, 3 = fair, 4 = poor, and 5 = very poor. Then initial the box at the bottom of your column. Add any comments about the child's behavior today on the back of this card.

Behaviors to be rated:	Class periods/subjects						
	1	2	3	4	5	6	7
Class participation							
Performance of class work							
Follows classroom rules							
Gets along well with other children							
Quality of homework, if any given							
Teacher's initials							

Place comments on back of card

DAILY SCHOOL BEHAVIOR REPORT CARD

Child's name_____ **Date**_____

Teachers:
Please rate this child's behavior today in the areas listed below. Use a separate column for each subject or class period. Use the following ratings: 1 = excellent, 2 = good, 3 = fair, 4 = poor, and 5 = very poor. Then initial the box at the bottom of your column. Add any comments about the child's behavior today on the back of this card.

	Class periods/subjects						
Behaviors to be rated:	1	2	3	4	5	6	7
Teacher's initials							

Place comments on back of card

-------------------------- Cut here after photocopying --------------------------

DAILY SCHOOL BEHAVIOR REPORT CARD

Child's name_____ **Date**_____

Teachers:
Please rate this child's behavior today in the areas listed below. Use a separate column for each subject or class period. Use the following ratings: 1 = excellent, 2 = good, 3 = fair, 4 = poor, and 5 = very poor. Then initial the box at the bottom of your column. Add any comments about the child's behavior today on the back of this card.

	Class periods/subjects						
Behaviors to be rated:	1	2	3	4	5	6	7
Teacher's initials							

Place comments on back of card

From *Defiant Children* (2nd ed.): *A Clinician's Manual for Assessment and Parent Training* by Russell A. Barkley. Copyright 1997 by The Guilford Press. Reprinted in *Your Defiant Child: Eight Steps to Better Behavior* by Russell A. Barkley and Christine M. Benton. Permission to photocopy this form is granted to purchasers of *Your Defiant Child* for personal use only (see copyright page for details).

DAILY RECESS AND FREE TIME BEHAVIOR REPORT CARD

Child's name_____ Date_____

Teachers:
Please rate this child's behavior today during recess or other free time periods in the areas listed below. Use a separate column for each recess/free time period. Use the following ratings: 1 = excellent, 2 = good, 3 = fair, 4 = poor, and 5 = very poor. Then initial at the bottom of the column. Add any comments on the back.

Behaviors to be rated:	Recess and free time periods				
	1	2	3	4	5
Keeps hands to self; does not push, shove					
Does not tease others; no taunting/put-downs					
Follows recess/free time rules					
Gets along well with other children					
Does not fight or hit; no kicking or punching					
Teacher's initials					

Place comments on back of card

------------------------- Cut here after photocopying -------------------------

DAILY RECESS AND FREE TIME BEHAVIOR REPORT CARD

Child's name_____ Date_____

Teachers:
Please rate this child's behavior today during recess or other free time periods in the areas listed below. Use a separate column for each recess/free time period. Use the following ratings: 1 = excellent, 2 = good, 3 = fair, 4 = poor, and 5 = very poor. Then initial at the bottom of the column. Add any comments on the back.

Behaviors to be rated:	Daily recess and free time periods				
	1	2	3	4	5
Keeps hands to self; does not push, shove					
Does not tease others; no taunting/put-downs					
Follows recess or free time rules					
Gets along well with other children					
Does not fight or hit; no kicking or punching					
Teacher's initials					

Place comments on back of card

From *Defiant Children* (2nd ed.): *A Clinician's Manual for Assessment and Parent Training* by Russell A. Barkley. Copyright 1997 by The Guilford Press. Reprinted in *Your Defiant Child: Eight Steps to Better Behavior* by Russell A. Barkley and Christine M. Benton. Permission to photocopy this form is granted to purchasers of *Your Defiant Child* for personal use only (see copyright page for details).

(cont. from p. 204)

- Has materials needed for class activities
- Finishes in-class assignments
- Follows directions
- Does work neatly
- Finishes tests
- Looks over work before handing in tests

Negative behaviors to discourage

- Hits, pushes, or bullies others
- Destroys school or class property (writing in textbooks, ruining play equipment, etc.)
- Interrupts the teacher/talks without being called on
- Leaves assigned seat/classroom/playground without permission
- Swears or uses obscenities
- Teases, insults, or picks on other children
- Is excessively noisy
- Is overly silly—the class clown

Reviewing the Report Cards at Home

Set up a regular routine for reviewing the cards with your child as soon as possible after school every day. When your child produces the card, *always begin by praising the child for any good ratings (1's and 2's).* Extending the "praise first" principle to school will encourage the good behavior that the teachers report to you. Only after you've done this should you discuss, in a neutral, businesslike fashion, any poor ratings (4's and 5's). As Janet and Jack did in the "after" scenario at the beginning of this chapter, ask your child what led to this poor behavior, but move on if your child begins to indulge in a long harangue or whining litany about the injustice of it all. Make it clear that the teacher's rating, based on his or her fair observations, is what you will rely on, not your child's excuses or any blaming of others for the child's behavior. Now add or subtract chips or tokens for the ratings on the card, according to the following scale—points for 8- through 12-year-olds, chips for 4- through 7-year-olds:

- 1 = +25 points/+5 chips
- 2 = +15 points /+3 chips
- 3 = +5 points/+1 chip
- 4 = –15 points/–3 chips
- 5 = –25 points/–5 chips

Add up the points for the positive ratings, subtract the penalties for the negative ratings, and add the total to, or subtract it from, the child's earnings for the day from home and public behaviors. Let the child use the day's total for privileges as always.

Trouble Spots and Stumbling Blocks

"The teacher is so skeptical about whether any new attempt to manage my son's behavior will be worth her time that she's not even willing to meet with me to discuss the idea. What can I do?"

First, try explaining to her that this program really relies more on you than on the teacher. All the teacher need do is record behavior ratings—a matter of a couple of minutes a day—and leave the consequences to you. Point out that if your son's behavior is that bad, undoubtedly she is already spending a lot of time paying attention to what he's doing, so no extra vigilance should be necessary.

Ask the teacher if she's willing to try the program for just a week on the understanding that she'll reconsider if she notices an improvement in your son's behavior by Friday.

If she won't budge, consider talking to the school psychologist or a guidance counselor. It's possible that this teacher doesn't have the time to devote much attention to individual behavior management or that she doesn't have the educational background to understand the potential gain. She may be more open to a request from another education professional.

If the teacher absolutely refuses to cooperate, you may still be able to implement this program in part by giving rewards for the behavior that you're already being informed about: points for Wnot getting a phone call from the teacher for a certain number of days; another number of points for not getting a note about the child's behavior; and so forth. If your child's school has a discipline program that includes, say, detention for behavioral infractions and rule violations, you can

penalize the child for each detention or reward him for every predes-
ignated time interval that goes by without a detention.

*"What do we do about a teacher who sends home report cards with all 4's and
5's all the time?"*

I assume you believe those ratings are unfair, in which case you
have to use your judgment. If your objection to those ratings stems
from your child's protests of innocence, talk to the teacher and ask for
details of the misbehavior. The success of this step depends on consistency and fairness from everyone involved. Perhaps the teacher is being a bit overzealous out of the belief that a bad report card will be a
faster, stronger motivator for change from your child. You now know
firsthand that positive reinforcement works better than excessive punishment. If you can do so tactfully, you might explain the parallels in
your home program that illustrate this point. If not, just gently suggest
that you add a behavior to the card that your child will easily do well
with so that she'll be motivated to keep working at her school behavior. If the teacher refuses and seems unreasonable, go to the school
principal for help.

*"Jimmy's teacher says she fills out enough forms already. She wants to help
but would rather just give us an informal report every day. Should we agree
to this?"*

You can, but it may be difficult to establish consistent and fair
consequences unless there's a systematic way of rating your child's behavior. We sometimes recommend a journal rather than the report
cards. In these cases, a steno-type notebook or spiral notebook goes
back and forth between parent and teacher, with each writing notes
about how the child is doing in that setting and any queries they have
for each other.

*"My daughter is doing everything she can to fight us on this—including not
bringing home her report card at all. What should we do?"*

You have to impose a significant penalty for not bringing home
the report card. Some parents find it sufficient to fine the child a total

equivalent to the worst possible report card ratings. Others ground the child for the day, cutting her off from all privileges that ordinarily can be bought via the token system.

"Katie is really used to getting chips immediately following good behavior and seems to be having trouble connecting what she did at preschool with the chips I give her when she gets home, so we're seeing the same pattern of ratings every day. In other words, we're making little progress. Any ideas?"

For some kids, consequences involving the token system simply are too distant to provide an incentive. Before you try anything else, though, are you remembering to offer praise and positive attention for reported good behavior the minute the child gets home? For many kids, that does the trick. If it's not enough for your daughter, try setting up a more tangible system of rewards, including a favorite snack right after school, extra TV time, a trip to the petting zoo for a whole week of good ratings, and so forth.

"My child is doing too well with this program. He's earning so many points that he can barely spend them all on privileges. What should we change?"

I've heard this before. Some kids notice their newfound wealth so quickly that they stop trying to earn points outside of school, and their home behavior plummets. The best thing to do in this case is to reevaluate how much each reward or privilege on the child's list costs. Then either add some new privileges so that the child needs more points to redeem them or raise the cost of the existing rewards so there's motivation to earn more points every day.

"My daughter's biggest problem is forgetting to write down her homework assignments. She's improved in every other area but that, and we're pretty much out of ideas. Help!"

Try using the back of the report card as an assignment log. Ask the teacher to have your child write the assignments on the back of the card as the day goes on. After each period, the teacher should check the assignment for accuracy before rating the child's behavior and initialing the card. Then, when the child gets home, you know that you and the child have an accurate record of the homework to be done.

"I'm suspicious. Suddenly my son is getting 1's and 2's on everything. Is that likely?"

Well, it's certainly possible, but since behavioral change is usually gradual, it's not too probable. I hate to say it, but kids have been known to take advantage of substitute teachers and other loophole opportunities to enter their own ratings and forge their teachers' initials. That's one reason you need to schedule meetings with the teacher—a perfect time to show the teacher the report cards and find out whether she in fact filled them out herself.

"Why does my daughter repeat the same mistakes several days in a row, despite having seen what the consequences are?"

The biggest impediment to benefiting from these report cards is the time lag between the school behavior and the consequences imposed at home. Some kids, especially if they have attentional problems like those that accompany ADHD, have trouble maintaining the behavior–consequence link, and it takes additional reinforcement—sometimes making the same mistake and suffering the same consequence several times—to make it stick. Sometimes it's the difference in surroundings that breaks the mental connection kids need to motivate themselves to behave well. Discussing with your child how she might handle a problematic situation differently tomorrow gives her a plan to follow, but can she hold on to that intention a day later, in the school setting? Many cannot, so I recommend that you remind your daughter of how she should behave in those situations right before sending her off to school.

"My son's teacher says he's really improving in the classroom, but the minute he gets to the playground he seems to let loose, and all rules are off. Why isn't the report card motivating him then?"

All kids need to let off steam at recess. It's not unusual for well-behaved children to have an occasional problem during this free period. For your son, the problem could be the change of scene: With less structure, he just forgets about the rules. Ask the teacher to use the "think ahead, think aloud" procedure before recess: The teacher should remind your child of the recess rules, note that they are listed on the report card, remind the child that he is being watched by the playground monitor, and tell the child to give the card to the monitor.

CHAPTER 12

Step 8:
Moving toward a
Brighter Future

The last step in our program represents a giant leap for parents of defiant children. This is where we send you off on your own, toward a future full of promise for your child and your family. By now you should have plenty of evidence that the last few months have been time well spent, that what you've learned together has benefits that reach far beyond the walls of your home. Getting along better with you naturally helps your child get along better with others. Being able to behave appropriately and follow rules at home gives your son or daughter the confidence and competence to lead a successful life in the wider world. You should now be able to look to the future with renewed hope that your child's tendency toward difficult behavior does not have to stand in the way of achieving a happy and healthy adulthood.

That does not mean that your job is over. You can withdraw the token systems and school behavior report cards that have supported your efforts so far—this chapter will show you how to do so wisely—but your parenting should be guided by the principles woven throughout this program forever. It's far too easy, many parents have found, to lapse back into negative old habits in dealing with a child who leans toward defiance. One important goal of this final step, then, is to give you a method for reviewing your own behavior when your child's behavior seems to go downhill.

Where Are You Now?

Assuming that you have spent at least two months on Steps 1–7 and that you stuck with each step as long as was necessary to see some improvement, your relationship with your child should now be on a somewhat even keel. At the very least some degree of lasting peace should have descended over your former battleground. To see how far you've come, fill out the forms on pages 7–8, 16–17, and 29–30 once again and compare them to the ones you filled out at the beginning of the program. If the forms don't show a significant improvement in your child's behavior now that you've completed Steps 1–7, please continue using all the techniques you've learned until you believe things are changing for the better. Then fill out the forms again to see if they agree. Generally, we consider improvement to be a reduction of scores in the range of 30 to 50% from your earlier scores. If you haven't gotten that far, stay on the program a little longer. I would also suggest that you persist for another month of the program if you've seen no change in the first two months. If by then nothing has changed, seek professional assistance for your child.

Next, turn back to page 33. Did the form you filled out there indicate that there was a chance your child has ADHD? If so, your child may need supports like the home token system for a long time and may also benefit from some other treatment, such as medication. Now is a good time to consider consulting a professional (see Chapter 3) if you haven't already done so and if your child can't seem to do without the incentives of tokens and the consistent use of penalties and time-out.

If, on the other hand, you have seen significant improvement in your child's behavior, you can try phasing out these supports.

Graduating from Tokens, Fines, and Report Cards

If your child is currently using the daily school behavior report card system, you will have to continue using the home token system as well, even if your child doesn't seem to need that incentive for good behavior at home. Your first goal, then, is to phase out the report card system.

Consider weaning your child from the report card program once he or she has two full weeks of school with no 4's or 5's on the report cards. At that point, ask the teacher to fill out the cards only on Wednesdays, reporting on behavior from Monday through Wednesday, and Fridays, reporting on Thursday and Friday behavior. Once your son or daughter completes another two weeks without any 4's or 5's, you can have the teacher switch to Fridays only, with the card reporting on the whole week's behavior. Another two weeks without a 4 or 5 means it's time to consider discontinuing the card. If you have seen your child improve at school because of some behavior modification technique, only to deteriorate again later, it would be wise to use monthly report cards for a while before phasing them out altogether. Otherwise, you can just check with the teacher monthly by phone.

Be sure to tell your child that eliminating the report cards does not mean the teacher will no longer pay attention to the child's behavior. In fact, if you get any negative reports from the teacher about your son or daughter's behavior, you will reinstitute the daily report cards.

Once your child is behaving acceptably at school without a behavior report card, you can consider cutting out the home token system on which the report cards depend. Assuming your child has been behaving well at home, tell him or her that you're going to suspend the token system for a few days and see how things go. You'll still be watching the child's behavior, of course, and you should also assure the child that receiving privileges will still be based on the child's behaving well. The only thing that will be missing is the recording of points or the accumulation of chips. As with the school system, if your child's behavior worsens without the formal home token system, simply reinstate it.

Heading Off Trouble by Knowing Your Child

Falling back on the home token system is not your only recourse when your child reverts to old misbehavior or comes up with some new manifestation of defiance. In fact, immediately resorting to the token system may not be the best response to emerging trouble. First, try to determine *why* your child is acting up again.

With all the changes they encounter as they grow, it's not unusual for children to face periodic challenges that they cannot meet with their newfound equanimity. To help both of you surmount these challenges as quickly and painlessly as possible, know your child and what's going on in his or her life. That is, *pay attention!* It's easy to let your guard down once you believe your child's behavior is under control, but remember that a child's environment is never fully under control. Peer pressures, promotion from grade to grade and school to school, physical maturation, and other facts of children's evolving lives demand your vigilance and your understanding. Watch what's happening in your child's world and anticipate problems based on what you already know about your child's strengths and weaknesses. *Think ahead and think aloud!*

You already use this important tool when major transitions are coming up in your child's daily life—when overnight guests are arriving, a party is scheduled, the family is going out to dinner, and so forth—but you can also use it when more major changes are expected. Is your son about to enter a new school for the first time in his life? Is your daughter's best friend moving out of town? Is your child's teacher being replaced in the middle of the year?

Don't limit your thinking ahead to those changes that affect your son or daughter directly. Remember that changes affecting the rest of the family or other parts of the child's world tend to trickle down to him as well. Are you and your spouse beginning to have marital problems or considering a separation? Are you expecting a new baby? Has anyone in the family developed a chronic illness? Are you starting a new job or going back to school?

Also remember that it's not only the so-called negative changes that can be stressful to your child. A parent's big job promotion, a move to a new, larger house, a transition to the "gifted" group in fourth grade, or a gift of a puppy from Grandma can throw your child into a tizzy the same way household conflict or some loss or disappointment can.

Besides anticipating the effect of major transitions in your child's life, be aware of situations and activities that are typically aggravating to him or her. If you've been paying attention, you already have a mental running list of these trouble spots; but in the name of thoroughness, when you have a minute, go back through the forms you filled out in Chapters 1 and 2 to identify areas that are particularly troublesome for your child. Make lists of places, situations, people, or other factors that often trigger defiance in your child. Engrave these trouble spots on your brain and resolve to think ahead and think aloud to head off problems when these factors inevitably enter your child's sphere. The box below lists typical trouble spots that other parents have identified for their children.

ANTICIPATING PROBLEMS

The following problem situations have been reported by numerous parents over the years. Perhaps some of them apply to your child, too.

• *Prolonged waits.* "Sitting still quietly for any length of time is always a problem for Ted," his father reported, "so we arm ourselves with plenty of absorbing activities and plan for extra rewards for his patience whenever we have to go to a doctor's or dentist's office or even wait in line for a popular movie. If we see long lines at the checkout when we go into the supermarket, we try to come back to shop later. I always have a little bag of chocolate-covered raisins in my pocket, which Ted loves, as rewards for every five minutes of patient waiting when we're taken by surprise and can't get out of waiting for something."

• *Making a new friend.* "I know there's potential for trouble whenever Darrell comes home and starts talking nonstop about a new friend he's made. When he really wants to impress someone, he always goes overboard and starts getting aggressively bossy, so we do our best to 'think aloud' and gently remind him of the rules in getting along with people—no shoving, no name calling, and so forth. Darrell really likes 'what if' games, so we sometimes come up with little scenarios to help him anticipate trouble himself: 'What if Danny came over to play and he asked if he could try out your new bike? What would you do?'"

• *Crowded social events.* "Teresa does pretty well one on one, and she's generally OK when there's an even number of girls so they can pair up (three is usually a problem), but she can really fall apart in a

(cont.)

---

big, uncontrolled group. Class time is fine because of the structure, but Brownies just didn't work for her. We hate to have her miss out on all these fun activities, though, so now we try to talk to the adults who are supervising and see if there's a way to draw Teresa out of the crowd for a breather every now and then during the activity. A little break often helps her avoid getting too wound up."

• *Company's coming.* "Tia never adjusts easily to changes in her routine, like having overnight guests in the house. We tried setting up a single set of 'company's coming' rules for these frequent occasions—both Mark and I have large families scattered all over the country—but after a while we realized Tia's misbehavior is different depending on who's visiting. When it's her grandparents, she falls back into wheedling and tantrums because she knows they're softies and will give in to a lot of her demands. When it's her cousins, she's more likely to get bossy, even physical, with them. So now we have separate sets of company rules, and we concentrate hard on a couple of behaviors in each: We give lots of points for not hitting or bossing the other kids when cousins are here—and take away lots for violations—and we assign lots of points to 'no begging' and 'no foot stamping' with grandparents. We let a lot of the other stuff slide, and most visits come off pretty smoothly."

• *Changes in work schedules.* "When I decided to go back to nursing after Max started school, we all had to adjust a little, but even Max seemed to settle in. Now, with the crunch the hospital is feeling, we're all filling in where we're needed and my schedule changes every three weeks. The first time I had to work part of the evening, I came home to what looked like a battlefield—clothes and toys everywhere, Max sitting in the time-out chair in tears, and my husband, Jeff, sitting in a chair in the family room gripping a drink like it was some life-saving elixir.

"When this situation continued the next evening and the next, Jeff and I finally decided we had to do something about it, so we sat down and had a family conference. When we asked Max gently but firmly what was going on ('What's been bothering you, honey?' rather than 'Why in the world are you behaving so badly?'—which is always a bad idea with Max), he told us he thought I was trying to get away from him because I didn't want to play with him anymore. I felt awful—I'd gotten so wrapped up in trying to manage my new crazy schedule that I'd for-
(cont.)

gotten all about special times with Max. Well, it took a little more than just making sure to schedule them in again. Max was still suspicious, waiting for me to slip up, so we had to do a little extra to convince him of our good faith. First, we made a big special-times schedule on an erasable board, and, as soon as I got my work schedule for the next three weeks, we filled in special times for each day. We included a column next to each day so that we could check off every special time we spent together. Then, for any that had to be put off for whatever reason, we had a box at the bottom of the schedule for rain checks. Every rain check had to be made up on my next days off, and for every three or more rain checks in a week, Max got to choose from a list of special activities outside the home that we would do together. The fact that we took all this trouble made him realize how much we cared, and the board was a great visual reminder."

• **Giving the child new responsibilities.** "One day, after Lakeshia had done such a great job putting away her toys, I made the mistake of announcing blithely that I thought she was old enough to start making her bed every day. Well, you would have thought I'd told her she was going to have to quit school and go work in a sweatshop. She turned on me and started screaming about how unfair I was and how she wasn't going to do it and I couldn't make her. I was so stunned I just backed off, but then James and I started talking about how we were going to make sure she took on new chores as she got older, as her brother and sister had.

"First we zeroed in on two mistakes I'd made: I hadn't told her first that she had done a terrific job of cleaning up the toys—that is, I hadn't praised her for what she'd just accomplished. I also hadn't made making her bed sound like a good thing—a responsibility she had earned for being so mature—so she thought it was some kind of punishment. Finally, I had forgotten one of the cardinal rules of living with Lakeshia: Give her some warning and build up slowly to changes in her routine. The solution was pretty simple. We talked to the older kids, who agreed to help us compliment Lakeshia for all the chores she was doing so responsibly these days, and we kept up a running dialogue about how if she kept this up she might be almost big enough to do things that Kenneth and Hannah could already do. By the time three weeks had passed, Lakeshia was practically begging us to teach her how to make

(cont.)

her bed, and she's been making it ever since—especially since one of us poked a head into her room while she was at it the first week to tell her what a great job she was doing."

• ***The arrival of a new baby.*** "I thought I knew what to expect from sibling rivalry since I already had two kids, but I am *so* glad our group talked about how new babies affect defiant children. The preparations I was able to make based on their experiences really helped what I now see could have been a pretty harrowing transition period for Dana. First, I vowed that special times would be sacrosanct, and I had a nice cuddle with Dana where I promised that we'd always have a special time together, even if it meant doing it while I kept the sleeping baby in a Snugli.

"We also talked about how frustrating new babies might seem and came up with a short list of new household rules regarding our new addition: 'No yelling at the baby,' 'no hitting the baby,' and 'no entering the baby's room when the baby is sleeping.' For the first month, Dana would get 5 extra points for obeying each of these rules for the day, and if she stuck to one of them for a whole week, she'd get 10 bonus points. To prevent arguments ('But, Mom, I didn't *know* the baby was sleeping') we agreed that we'd hang a sign on the nursery door with 'Zzzzz' on it as a signal that the baby was asleep.

"There have been moments when Dana has really acted up when the baby has been cranky and so have I, but in general our planning has really helped. The other day she said to me very solemnly that the baby could play with us during our special times if she wanted to. I thought that was pretty cute since she's only two months old, but I hid my smile and said back just as seriously, 'Thanks, honey, that's really generous of you, but I don't want anything to interfere with our special times together. They're just too important to me.'"

What to Do When Defiance Returns

"Think ahead/think aloud" means more than communicating the rules and the consequences for your child right before a transition takes place. It also means having a plan for how you will respond when your child starts misbehaving. Here is what we recommend:

1. When your child starts to misbehave repeatedly, take out a notebook or pad and record the details of the problem: what your child is doing wrong (what rule is being broken), when, where, and what you are doing to try to manage the behavior.

2. Keep this record for a week or so, recording both what is repeated in the child's behavior and what new twists turn up.

3. Now review your notebook to see if you can find clues about how *you* are "misbehaving." If you look at what has been happening honestly, you may very well find that the problem is being caused by—or aggravated by—your return to negative old ways of managing your child: overpunishing, coercing, asking for favors, being inconsistent, being unfair, or not being specific. As you look through your record, ask yourself the following questions. For any "yes" answers, reread the chapter in parentheses.

- Have I been repeating my commands too often before imposing a consequence for noncompliance? (Chapter 6)
- Have I been giving ineffective commands? (Review Step 2 if you don't remember exactly what these are.) (Chapter 6)
- Have I been forgetting to pay attention and praise my child for compliance? (Chapter 5)
- Have I been failing to provide rewards or privileges for obeying the rules and complying with commands? (If so, you've probably stopped the token system too soon and need to return to it until these habits are second nature.) (Chapter 7)
- Have I been postponing penalties or punishment until my child has forgotten what the consequence is for? (Chapters 8 and 9)
- Have I let the practice of special time together slide? (Chapter 5)

4. Now take action to correct your own behavior: Practice the techniques you've learned as reviewed and give yourself a couple of days to see if the problem begins to resolve itself.

5. If not, tell your child what you expect from him or her regarding the misbehavior that's occurring ("From now on, you may not leave your desk until your homework is finished"; "There will be no more swearing in the house"; "Snacks are not allowed to be eaten anywhere except the kitchen without permission from me or Dad") and set up a token system to reward compliance with the rule you've just explained. Be sure to pay close enough attention to give out tokens whenever they are earned.

6. Impose time-out every time the misbehavior is repeated from now on.

7. If your record shows that the misbehavior occurs in a particular setting, use the think ahead/think aloud system to resolve it (see Chapter 10).

8. Continue to take notes until the problem seems to have disappeared.

If none of this works, you may need professional help. See Chapter 3.

A Final Word

Congratulations! You've completed one of the most effective courses on child behavior management used by mental health counselors. If all went well, you have witnessed improvements in your relationship with your child, in your stress levels as a parent, and in your child's ability to fulfill responsibilities and meet others' expectations. You may even find that the benefits of the program have extended to your other children as well.

Most parents tell us that this program has left them with a new sense of their own competence and a new confidence that they are prepared to meet the future and any behavioral difficulties that might arise. You deserve a great deal of credit for the dedication and perseverance you have invested in this program, and you deserve the self-assurance you have earned. By doing your best to change yourself—in the ways you interact with your child and manage your child's behavior—you have encouraged your child to be more responsive to direction, more trustworthy in carrying out day-to-day responsibilities, and more positive and effective in interactions with others. And you can't do any better than that as a parent.

Appendix

Does Your Child Have Conduct Disorder?

If you answered "often" or "very often" to six or more of the questions in the first questionnaire in this book and/or if your child is violent, you should seek professional help. First, however, fill out the following form. If you answer "Yes" to three or more of these items, your child may have conduct disorder and should be evaluated as soon as possible.

Circle "Yes" for any behavior your child has engaged in over the last 12 months:

1. Often bullied, threatened, or intimidated others		No	Yes
2. Often initiated physical fights		No	Yes
3. Used a weapon that can cause serious physical harm to others (e.g., a bat, brick, broken bottle, knife, or gun)		No	Yes
4. Has been physically cruel to people		No	Yes
5. Has been physically cruel to animals		No	Yes
6. Has stolen while confronting a victim (e.g., mugging, purse snatching, extortion, armed robbery)		No	Yes
7. Has forced someone into sexual activity		No	Yes
8. Has deliberately engaged in fire setting with the intention of causing serious damage		No	Yes
9. Has deliberately destroyed others' property (other than fire setting)		No	Yes
10. Has broken into someone else's house, building, or car		No	Yes

11. Often lies to obtain goods or favors or to avoid obligations
    (i.e., "cons" others)   No   Yes

12. Has stolen items of value without confronting a victim
    (e.g., shoplifting without breaking and entering; forgery) No   Yes

13. Often stays out at night despite parental prohibitions   No   Yes
    If so, at what age did your child begin doing this? _____

14. Has run away from home overnight at least twice while
    living in parents' home, foster care, or group home   No   Yes
    If so, how many times? _____

15. Is often truant from school   No   Yes
    If so, at what age did he/she begin doing this? _____

Resources

Support Groups for Parents

Unfortunately, to date there are no support groups or other organizations dedicated specifically to defiance in children. Because so many defiant children have ADHD, I suggest you tap into the well-established network of support services for parents of children with ADHD. The national organizations will gladly refer you to the support group closest to you:

CHADD (Children with Attention Deficit Disorders) National Headquarters
499 Northwest 70th Ave.
Suite 109
Plantation, FL 33317
(305) 587-3700 or (800) 233-4050

CHADD is the largest national association for these disorders, currently having more than 500 local affiliates in almost every state.

ADDA (National Attention Deficit Disorder Association)
P.O. Box 972
Mentor, OH 44061
(800) 487-2282

If no support is available in your area, or you find that groups begun by parents of children with ADHD near you do not address defiance in enough depth, consider starting your own group. Many parents who have gone through the training program at our clinic have done just that, by putting out flyers announcing their intention and soliciting interested parents. Try leaving flyers at local schools, pediatricians' offices, and mental health clinics. You may be surprised by the number of responses you get; parents of defiant children are usually so relieved to have a venue for talking about their concerns that they are very open to participating.

On the Net

On-line resources grow in number seemingly every day, and they often disappear as quickly, so these addresses may not be accurate by the time you read this book. Search the Internet for new sources of information.

An on-line bulletin board for ADHD issues:

alt.support.attn-deficit

A website for CHADD's chapters:

www.chadd.org

Parent Training

How do you find a qualified therapist once you decide you would like to receive parent training from a professional? It is always sound advice to start by asking your child's pediatrician for referrals to professionals who conduct behavioral parent training programs. Also, if you expect your health insurance plan to cover any of the costs of professional services for your child, the plan may require that you contact your pediatrician first about such a referral.

You can also contact your local mental health clinic or association for referrals or contact your nearest university medical center and speak with someone in the child psychology or psychiatry service to see if professional services for defiant children or formal parent training programs are offered. If not, ask if there is anyone in the area they can recommend.

Your child's school may also be of some assistance. Speak to the school psychologist or social worker to see if he or she is familiar with professionals in the region who provide the sorts of services you are seeking, specifically this parent training program. Or call your school district headquarters and ask whether your district has a special education parent advisory committee. All school districts have a special education program, and most have a parent advisory committee connected with them. The parents on this committee can be a tremendous source of referrals.

As with finding a support group, however, your best bet may be to contact the national office of CHADD (address and phone number above) to find your local chapter and ask the local chapter for referrals. CHADD's strength is that it is an organization of parents like you, and other parents, you will find, are probably your greatest resource. These are the people who can direct you to the professionals who have a track record of providing real help to parents. When you call your CHADD contact, ask direct questions such as "Who is a good therapist in the area?" and "Who can help our family?" or "Who can help us as parents?"

If there is no CHADD chapter in your region, check your telephone directory for any other parent support organizations dedicated to ADHD children. Many parts of the country have freestanding, independent support groups that may not be affiliated with the CHADD organization yet can provide some information on mental health professionals in your area.

When you contact the professionals to whom you have been referred, don't hesitate to ask if the therapist is familiar with Dr. Russell Barkley's parent training program for defiant children. If not, ask if the therapist provides behavioral parent training programs. If this therapist does not, find out if he or she knows someone who does.

Once you do find a therapist who has been of help to you in resolving the problems discussed in this book, please pass on the information. Call your local CHADD chapter or any similar organization you've identified and share your experience so that you in turn can help other parents.

Suggested Reading

Some of the books in the following list provide more technical information than parents may wish to read. But for those of you who are interested in acquiring more detailed, scientific information on children's behavioral disorders, these titles offer some new insights. Many of these books can be found in large public or university libraries.

Barkley, R. A. (1995). *Taking charge of ADHD: The complete, authoritative guide for parents.* New York: Guilford Press.

Barkley, R. A. (1997). *Defiant children* (2nd ed.)*: A clinician's manual for assessment and parent training.* New York: Guilford Press.

Barkley, R. A. (1998). *Attention-deficit hyperactivity disorder: A handbook for diagnosis and treatment* (2nd ed.). New York: Guilford Press.

Campbell, S. B. (1990). *Behavior problems in preschool children.* New York: Guilford Press.

Forgatch, M., & Patterson, G. R. (1990). *Parents and adolescents living together.* Eugene, OR: Castalia.

Hinshaw, S. P. (1994). *Attention deficits and hyperactivity in children.* Thousand Oaks, CA: Sage.

Hinshaw, S. P., & Anderson, C. A. (1996). Conduct and oppositional defiant disorders. In E. J. Mash & R. A. Barkley (Eds.), *Child psychopathology* (pp. 113–152). New York: Guilford Press.

Latham, P., & Latham, R. (1992). *ADD and the law.* Washington, DC: JKL Communications.

Mash, E.J., & Barkley, R. A. (Eds.). (1996). *Child psychopathology.* New York: Guilford Press.

Mash, E. J., & Barkley, R. A. (Eds.). (1998). *Treatment of childhood disorders* (2nd ed.). New York: Guilford Press.

Weiss, G., & Hechtman, L. T. (1993). *Hyperactive children grown up: ADHD in children, adolescents, and adults* (2nd ed.). New York: Guilford Press.

Index

Stress
  as causes of recent changes in
    behavior, 12–13
  family, when to seek help, 89
  financial and occupational
    problems, 44
  marital discord, 44, 67–68
  parent's, dealing with, 68
  personal and health problems, 44
  relationships with others, 44
  single parent, 43–44
Success of program, case example,
  64–67
Support group
  benefits of, 59–60
  locating, 59
  resources for, 227–228

T

Talk during special time
  technique, 100–102
Tantrums. *See* Temper tantrums
Tasks, targeting for rewards, 135,
  139, 143
Tattling and punishment, 168
Teacher. *See also* School setting
  daily behavior report card,
    200–204
  enlisting aid of, 60–61
  unwillingness to meet with parent,
    209–210
Telephone calls
  reducing interruptions, 118–120,
    123, 125, 127
  right and wrong way to handle,
    121–122
Temper tantrums
  anticipating with punishment
    program, 154–155
  on way to or in time-out, 162
Temperament of child
  clashing with that of parent,
    34–35
  effects on behavior, 31–32
  factor in determining behavior,
    25
  rating, 29–31
  recognizing what can be changed
    and what can't, 61–64

Tests
  Behavior in Various School
    Situations, 202
  Could Your Child Have ADHD?,
    33
  Defiance in Various Home
    Situations, 16–17
  Profile of Family Problems, 45–46
  Profile of Your Characteristics,
    35–36
  Profile of Your Child's
    Temperament, 29–31
  simple behavior frequency, 7–8
Therapist
  characteristics of good, 51–52
  parent training, selecting for,
    228–229
  types of treatment, 58
  when to seek help, 3, 13, 14
Time involvement
  special time technique, 104–105
  teacher, 209–210
  token program, 147
Time lag for consequences
  public places to home, 195–196
  school setting to home, 212
Time-out
  acting out behavior, 157–160
  alternatives to chair, 162–163, 181
  apologizing after, 181
  avoiding penalty, 177
  behavior not targeted for, 166
  car, using in, 195
  case example, 171–172
  child not complying after, 178
  child's reaction to, 176–177
  complaints of unfairness, 182
  description of, 86
  duration of, 158
  exceptions to procedure, 159
  household rules and, 159,
    178–179
  leaving without permission,
    161–165, 180–181
  misbehavior during, 176
  parental conflict over punishment,
    180
  prior use of, 166
  procedures for, 157–159
  public, using in, 191–192, 193
  reviewing progress, 172–176